CW00503861

Make or *Break*

The Extraordinary Life of Paul Innes

PAUL INNES

Queensland, Australia

Copyright © 2022 by Paul Innes

All rights reserved. Apart from fair dealing for the purposes of study, research, criticism or review as permitted under the Copyright Act, no part of this publication may be reproduced, distributed or transmitted in any form or by any means without prior written permission.

The information in this book is not intended to replace professional medical or psychological advice. The content is based upon the author's personal and professional experiences, opinions and qualifications.

All necessary written permissions have been obtained from others to publish their stories. Some names have been changed to protect identities, whereas others have asked that their real names be used.

www.independenceworld.com.au

Cover design by Judith San Nicolas
Typeset in Garamond 9/12pt & Abadi Extra Light 22pt
Printed and bound in Australia by IngramSpark
Prepared for publication by Dr Juliette Lachemeier @ The Erudite Pen

NATIONAL
LIBRARY
OF AUSTRALIA

A catalogue record for this book is available from the National Library of Australia

Make or Break: The Extraordinary Life of Paul Innes — 1st edition
ISBN Paperback - 9780645600506
ISBN Ebook - 9780645600513

Dedication

To the most selfless person I have ever known, my footy rival, my punting partner and my best mate – my mum. Without your dedication, this book would have only been a dream.

CONTENTS

Preface 1

A Somewhat Industrious Boy 3

The Neighbourly Demon & the Fire Ring 11

My Profound Candle Stare 13

The Green Border & Fake Honesty Box 15

Through the Bull to Get to the Gold 19

Cross-Dressing & Croc Surfing 25

Strangulation by Uncertain Burton 27

Inmates of the Lost World 39

Mafia Thriller Stripper 41

Jive Dude Turkey 43

My Gypsie 47

The Beaming Preacher 51

My Life Changes Forever 55

Why the Channel 7 Chopper Chills Me to My Feet 59

My Angel Flies Free 69

Medication or Meditation? 73

Bringing the SWAT Team to Their Knees 83

The Mary Poppins Stunt 89

In Spirit & in Truth 93

Squashing My Balls 97

The Appreciation Celebration 101

The Natural Love Sanctuary 109

An Ashram in India..119

The Sanctuary Becomes Self-Sufficient.............................125

The LSD Hitman...139

Australia's First Rainbow Gathering....................................143

Off-the-Grid Treasures...151

My Friends are Frogs..159

Tie His Schlong to His Leg..165

Backwards Walked the Black Witch....................................169

Scratching My Neck..173

Voicing Peace of Mind..177

An Ocean of Emotion...181

Trying to be Normal..185

The Crazy With Pink Earrings...191

The Phoenix Jack...195

The Night Job..197

The Rollover of the Standover..205

Taking Care of Business...209

Happy Paul..219

The Pursuit of Understanding & Change............................223

I Hope My Karma Doesn't Run Over My Dogma.................229

The Future, The Present & Staying Pleasant.......................233

Lucid Dreams Are Not What They Seem.............................237

My Best Mate...247

A Delight to Write...Not My Last Chapter...........................249

Acknowledgements..257

Preface

I have written this autobiography to illuminate the power, true beauty and genuine freedom of our spirit, and to highlight the strength and fulfilment that comes from community support.

From the gangs on the streets of Western Sydney, sustaining a life-changing injury, becoming a self-sufficient community founder and frog defender to a rights advocate, sit-down comedian, ghost hunter and forming my band, my life has been a pretty extreme but insanely cool rock and rollercoaster ride.

May this book serve to invigorate and empower you as an individual, to dream unbounded and to draw the infinite power of life out of every living moment.

A Somewhat Industrious Boy

BOOSH! The ground shook as splinters of wood and smoke bellowed above the tree line in the distance. There was yelling in the camp like, 'They've blown themselves up!' 'The army will have heard that one!' 'They'll think we're the Japs. Run!' as we all took flight in the general direction of the road. Some of these boys I did not know well, and they seemed like they enjoyed the obvious danger. After what seemed like only seconds of silence following the explosion, the whirring of helicopter blades and the roar of multiple vehicle engines could be heard. A machine gun fired off in the distance at an unknown target, and as we were right on the outskirts of an army base, this explosion meant business. We were in big trouble.

We lived in St Marys, a suburb of western Sydney. For a bunch of young teenagers in 1981, we were pretty mischievous, but until now our fun always seemed mostly harmless. It was a regular activity for us on the weekends to tell our parents we were sleeping over at a friend's place. They too were friends and never checked with each other, so we were able to sneak out. This enabled us to make our way past the grumpy old farmer on his land at the edge of where the local industrial estate began, through the wet and slippery pitch-black underground drains, shuffle under the barbed wire fence, slowly crawl past the civilian army compound and eventually into the scrub of the ammunition dump, where we would camp for the weekend. The camp was made out of old materials taken from the army sheds, and even made a rickety raft out of a few planks tied down to two 44-gallon drums.

The trouble started when on one weekend of exploring, we stumbled across another shed filled with gelignite explosives. Previously, we'd played with modified firecrackers, which wouldn't do too much damage, except for a few destroyed letter boxes. We quickly worked out how to set off the gelignite through knowledge gained from the movies we'd watched. Since finding the gelignite, we had only blown up some trees and little objects with small amounts of the explosive. It took a few weekends before our supply had run out. The older boys decided to go out to look for more, and the big explosion was the next thing that followed.

Wazza was one of my closest mates, and he and I hightailed it until we were way in front of all the rest. We had been running for about five minutes when we hid behind some trees and looked back. Two of the kids I had grown up with, Jackson and Bulldog, were being herded into the back of an army jeep with the barrel of a gun at their back. With our hearts racing and adrenaline pumping, we took off again and managed to make it all the way to the edge of the farm. We rested by the farmer's dam, just metres from the road, to catch our breath. The army no longer seemed to be after us, so I smugly declared that we had successfully escaped.

'Don't look now, Innes, but the farmer has a double-barrel at the back of your head,' said Wazza with a smirk.

'Bulls**t,' I said as I laughed.

'I'll bet you your new pocketknife,' he countered.

I turned slowly, only to see the two dark holes of the gun sitting betwixt my eyes, and behind them the furrowed, menacing scowl of the farmer. A sense of dread came over me as I accepted defeat. He rounded us up and escorted us to the police station, just to the side of the civilian army compound.

Between the army, the police and the farmer, we were all eventually captured. Being reunited again at the police station, I looked around and saw a couple of faces full of regret and worry, and others that were more indignant. Some of the older boys were true rebels, unlike me, and had been in trouble with the police before. As the police sat us down by their desks and started interrogations, the older boys demanded they be given food and drink. I could not believe it when the police bowed to their demands, going to the shop and bringing back an assortment of goods. I was astounded at the cheek of the boys but had to admire their nerve. As the questions were fired, we vowed to stay silent, but the police told us we would not be leaving until we gave up our parents' phone numbers. After a few hours of stalling, we realised we had no choice.

I hoped that my usually sweet and forgiving mother would arrive and tell me that everything would be alright. After a long period of trepidation, my heart sank to see my father's car pull up. Dad was a big man and took no crap from anybody. He was dressed in his work clothes as the manager of the Penrith Panthers Leagues Club. His tie was flapping and his silver pocket pen glinting as he walked swiftly into the police station. Without a word, even though I was twelve years old, he picked me up and threw me over his shoulder like some sort of baggage. He then turned and headed straight back towards the door. A policeman, who was also rather large, blocked the door and declared I needed to be 'processed'.

Dad arced up and growled, 'You can't charge him, he's just a kid!' pushing the policeman with force to one side. We continued to the car, and they let us go.

An intense couple of minutes passed as Dad said nothing to me. I imagined he was so angry that he was saving his temper for when he pulled the car up at any moment to give me the belting of my life. I could not take it anymore. I conjured up a quick and weak lie that we just got lost while exploring. I opened my mouth and only managed to mutter the first word before he dismissed the incident as trivial. I was stunned. Though my misbehaviour was not a very regular occurrence, he'd had much stronger reactions to it before. Even the sound of his authoritative voice was usually enough to make me tremble.

As we opened the door to our house, I expected a cuddle from Mum and the soft words I was used to. Instead, a wooden rolling pin came flying at my head as she swung to get me! 'You little mongrel, bringing the coppers to our door!'

Dad ducked my head and pushed me inside, telling me I'd better get in my bedroom until she'd calmed down. What a role reversal! I later found out that the police had come during one of Mum's big card games. Mum's card games with her friends were one of her favourite pastimes. Regularly by the end of the night, the drinking and gambling deteriorated into a strip show on top of the kitchen table. One of Mum's best friends, Sheryl, had big boobs, and I was secretly in love with her. It was at the beginning of any strip show that we kids felt compelled to leave, which is when we were able to get up to our mischief and escape out to our campsite.

The western suburbs of Sydney were rough, where department houses stretched for tens of miles and children roamed in gangs. Originally being born in Darlinghurst in 1968, we had moved there from Redfern in the city when I was just two years of age. I was the youngest of three children in our family. My brother Danny was four years my senior, whom I loved playing cricket and football with, but he also enjoyed holding me down and spitting on me, which smelled like it came from a rotten corpse. My sister Debbie, nine years older than me, took care of me when Mum was busy or working.

When Danny was older, he got a job at the railway. He had to get up early when it was cold, so he grew an afro to keep himself warm, and I called him 'hair bear'. Debbie by then was working at the local store and had saved enough to go on a big cruise ship around the Pacific when she was only sixteen. She soon left home and settled in Far North Queensland at age eighteen. We cacked ourselves laughing when we saw a photo of her and realised that she had become a 'hippie'.

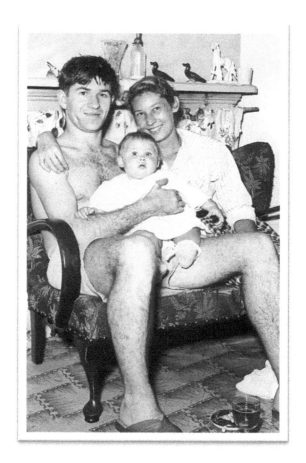

My Dad, Mum and Debbie in 1960.

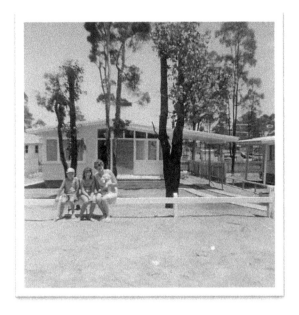

Danny, Deb and Mum outside our government house before
there were paths or lawn.

My mum, Josie, had always been a selfless person. She was
forever making sure everyone had eaten enough and was
warmly clothed. With her beautiful smile and cheery little
hum, she would make me feel relaxed and content while we
waited for a bus or train. Mum worked in catering at the Royal
Easter Show and other places like the cricket and races. Soon
after I was conceived, my father, Ray, and my mum separated,
and she was worried that she would not be able to handle or
afford a third child. Her friend knew a lady who could tell her
how to perform an abortion, so she set off to find out how.
Sunlight soap, a douche kit and the schnapps were ready when
her friend arrived back, frantically knocking on the door. She

had found out that somebody had died trying the same method. With that, Mum decided to have me. Nature has been trying to knock me off ever since.

Mum and Dad reconciled their differences and got back together before I was born. From the age of around twelve, I started working in the same places as Mum. I still remember the smell of the old wooden cricket stand and the small souvenir bats we would ask the cricket stars to sign. I also loved to go to work early in the morning with Dad sometimes, where he would let me play the 'one-armed bandits' or pokies. A somewhat industrious boy, I took every opportunity for work that presented itself, from the fruit juice run and delivering bags of oranges to a K-mart storeman.

I began writing very young and especially liked to write songs to entertain my friends. They would regularly ask me to sing them, and I was always happy to oblige. My schoolteachers encouraged me in entertainment, and I became the leading role in many school plays, even travelling with the school to perform at other schools in the area.

My family was middle-class, I suppose. I was well-loved and cared for and there was always plenty of food and pressies on special occasions. One of my treasured memories was visiting my Aunty Margo. She was always making me laugh with her one crazy-eye look. Her house smelled so clean, and she seemed rich because she wore gold. I soon realised that she had probably become rich through the money that she had saved from when we went for our early morning walks to steal the bread and paper.

The Neighbourly Demon & the Fire Ring

The resilience I relied on later on in life may have stemmed from one of my earliest memories. Glen, the boy next door, was only about a year older than me. He loved to taunt me and would regularly capture and terrorise me. His mother Sharon was a lovely lady, and she babysat me for a couple of years from the age of two. Though she was very sweet, one of my earliest memories was the vomit-like smell of the baby food Sharon fed me while in my highchair.

Though Glen and I did play together, it was more like he was just playing *with* me. I learned that I could never trust him, becoming acutely aware of my safety when he was around. One day, when I was about four years old, he led us both to a paddock only four doors away from where we lived. The grass in the paddock at the time was around three feet tall and completely dry from the scorching hot summer. Glen suggested we play a game. He asked me to sit down in the middle of the paddock and stay still. I was excited, thinking we were just playing a new game. He tried to keep out of sight, but I could just catch a glimpse of him as he walked in a circle around me, about twenty feet in radius. I soon heard crackling and saw some fire and smoke. Glen had been dropping matches in an apparent attempt to burn me alive!

Realising I was in grave danger and catalytic with fear, I began to scream and cry. Seemingly within no time at all, my hero appeared. It was a little old lady. Elsie lived at the end of the street and had heard me from her kitchen window. She casually picked me up and walked calmly back through the fire and smoke, into safety.

As an adult, experiences like this have helped me to appreciate that though the nature of some humans can be malicious, most people are indeed good-natured, and we always live on the edge of the fire of life and death.

My Profound Candle Stare

At the age of six, I did something that looking back now, I find profoundly useful in my adult life. I had been experiencing a tough time with the local kids as usual and sought solace in some way. Though our household was not religious as such, my mother did teach me to pray. One particular day, without being ever shown or asked to do, I began what became a regular ritual.

I set up a small table in our hallway. I placed a lit candle on it and shut all the doors so that it was now pitch dark except for the gently flickering flame. Sitting cross-legged in front of the table, I would stare at the candle, closing and opening my eyes ever so slowly until I could see the flame in my mind's eye just as well as I could see it with my eyes open.

As an adult, I have learned that this is a meditation technique used by many masters in the East, called Jyoti. It is used to develop the power of visualisation, strengthen photographic memory, build concentration skills and for the manifestation of co-creation. As I learned to hold the candlelight in my mind, thoughts tried to invade. Eventually, I could see them coming and was able to ignore them. This left me with the experience of just pure peace.

We are co-creators with the universe. It is our choice to create using the positive emotions of love, peace, freedom and joy, the thoughts of limitlessness and immortality, the words of wisdom, compassion and appreciation, and the actions of love, duty and service. Or to create with negative things like emotions of hatred, thoughts of vengeance, words of cursing or actions of violence, knowing repercussion or karma is magnified according to our choice.

The light of a candle is soft enough to gaze into without irritating your vision, and the element of fire is symbolic of the human condition, purifying everything in its golden flame. Jyoti has served me well throughout life, helping me to clear my mind when needed, to sharpen my focus on a task and to keep my brain sharp.

The Green Border & Fake Honesty Box

I was in my early teens when my sister's boyfriend Phil was involved in a car crash and received quite a bit of gravel rash along with a banged-up knee. I really looked up to him, so she took me to visit him after he had been in hospital for around three weeks. Phil told me that he had been saving something for me and handed me a jar. I looked at its contents with the jar close to my face and could not work out what it was. He then told me that it was the scabs he had collected as they had peeled off his wounds. It immediately sickened me in my stomach, and I nearly dropped the jar. I looked at him and he had a straight face. I felt obliged to humbly and meekly thank him for the gift.

He burst into laughter, and I realised the joke was on me. He then told me to hand them back because he was hungry. I never knew when he was joking but this one stuck with me. The perfect blend of a classic funny with the desired grossness for a young boy. Phil's dry 'dad jokes' paved the way for my own humour throughout life, with me now having told this story to many children.

Soon after, Dad decided to take my brother and me for a drive to Cairns for a holiday and to visit my sister, where she was now living. The journey from Sydney was long, and as a young boy, mostly boring to me. As we neared the end of our journey between Townsville and Cairns, we passed through the small town of Cardwell. On the outskirts, the environment turned unexpectedly lush. I had never seen such abundant and thick flora. We had truly entered a jungle. It was as though we had just passed a green border. The air smelled and felt different. The rainforest canopy formed an arch across some parts of the road. I could see scurrying wildlife and hear an orchestra of birds. Suddenly, I felt alive like never before. I was interested in everything.

As we drove along mesmerised by the diversity, I noticed a stall on the side of the road full of fruits I'd never seen before. There were vivid vegetables and brightly coloured bunches of flowers. That's when I noticed the sign that read 'Honesty Box'. I immediately laughed and relayed to my dad and brother that it was a set-up to catch thieves. Where I had come from, no such thing could possibly exist.

My dad began to explain that people were different in this part of the world and wanted to trust that others would be fair and do the right thing. I quickly dismissed his theory as old-school ignorance. We only got up the road about another mile when there was yet another stall with the same sign. I was stunned and silent. I wondered if we had entered a time warp or maybe a futuristic idealistic society. Maybe people here were so far away from the big city that they had never had reason not to trust each other. I eventually opted for the latter.

We arrived and stayed with my sister and Phil at their home on the foreshore of Machans Beach. Phil and I would get up at the crack of dawn and use the drag net just out from the beachfront to catch prawns. We caught bucketloads as big as bananas. In the mornings, we cooked them up for breakfast, and it was as though we were eating like royalty.

A couple of years after being back in Sydney, my brother Danny decided to move to Cairns to live with his girlfriend, Anne-Marie. Mum and Dad divorced when I was around age fourteen, and the next year in 1982, Mum and I followed my brother and sister north to settle in Cairns and its beautiful surrounds.

Through the Bull to Get to the Gold

The family needed money, so instead of going to school in Cairns, I began to look for a job. My first was at a fish and chip shop but then I decided to try something new. My sister's boyfriend Phil had been a big influence on my life. He had taught my brother Danny and me how to dangerous drive, or recover from a dangerous situation in a vehicle, before he taught us how to drive. He also showed us everything from growing tomatoes, rabbit shooting and preparing a reared chicken for the pot, to catching prawns, fixing cars and riding a motorbike. I realise now that I was very fortunate to have a strong male influence to look up to, with the patience to teach me many things about becoming an independent man as a lot of young people are not afforded this opportunity in life.

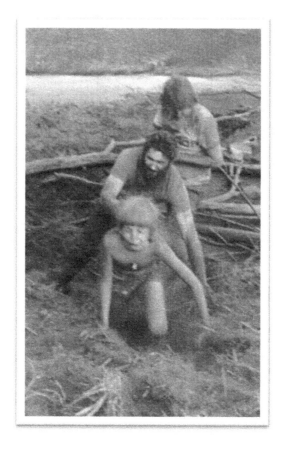

Phil chasing me while my brother tries to clean
his mouth in a dirt fight.

Phil suggested we try to make some money by hitchhiking from Cairns to Bowen to go tomato picking. I quickly agreed and packed my bags. We made it as far as Innisfail before the local police arrested us for hitchhiking. I said that Phil was my brother-in-law, but my sister and he were not married and did not have the same last name; therefore, and because I was only

20

a minor, they arrested us on suspicion that I was a runaway. They threw us in separate jail cells, and I gave them cheek. They eventually let Phil go without charge. I, however, was taken back to Cairns and made to sit in the office amongst many desks until my mum arrived.

Phil and I decided to try to look for work again. This time when we got to the highway, we headed north instead of south. Our best idea was to look for gold. Phil knew a man named Louie, who had a property at a place called Gold Hill, up the notorious CREB Track. The track was a single lane of dirt and mud through the rainforest from Daintree to Cooktown. It was made by the local electricity company to service their line. Louie needed help fixing his dozer so that he could move some rocks in a creek to look for gold, but most people found it too difficult to even get to the property. Phil rang his friend Gus, and they arranged to meet there and help Louie fix the dozer while also doing a bit of gold dredging and panning with Louie.

We hitched until we got to the Daintree Store. From there we walked the next few miles to the Daintree River Crossing without seeing another car. Around halfway there, I began to lag behind up to 50 metres. Out of the blue, I looked up to see a large herd of Brahman Bulls right across the road. Phil was standing on the other side! I panicked and yelled, 'What do I do?'

He told me to simply walk through them as they were docile. I did not believe him and froze. They were nearly as tall as me and there were about forty of them. He told me to hurry up or he would leave me behind. I had no choice and found I actually had to push some of them out of the way.

We arrived at the wide river crossing and contemplated our strategy. Soon enough, a convoy of four-wheel drives arrived on their way to Cooktown. They happily agreed to give us a lift. We rode in the first vehicle of the convoy, and they communicated with each other by walkie-talkie. Eventually, after navigating some treacherous trenches, we reached the bottom of a steep hill.

The driver stopped and told us that because the track was slippery, we would gun it until we reached the crest. No sooner had he put his foot down when an army convoy came over the top of the hill towards us. There were big trucks and there were plenty of them. It felt like we were in vehicular danger with the position we were in. It was better for us to just reverse back and out of the way. We parked just off the track at the bottom of the hill. One by one, each vehicle descended the hazardous track. A few had passed by when suddenly a jeep and trailer lost control and headed sideways down the hill, directly towards us. We leaped from our car into the jungle. Yet the driver somehow miraculously straightened up and gained control. We were very pleased when the last vehicle passed us.

Arriving at Gold Hill, Louie and his wife Megan were happy to see us and made us feel at home. We had a cup of tea and set up our camp not far from the main house. Early the next morning we woke and got ready for work. Phil and Gus looked to me as though they were fit men, and they both had big muscles. Louie asked them to carry a battery for the dozer to where it had broken down around a mile away. The battery was heavy, and the two of them had to take one side each. Louie stayed to talk with me for around ten minutes before he told me he needed to take the second battery also. Though Louie was a small man, he threw the battery on his shoulder and jogged away with it. Later they told me he passed them and laughed.

Louie shot a pig for dinner. For the next few days, we ate everything pig. No matter how many ways it was prepared, and there were many ways, it was delicious. We woke one morning ready to do some dredging and panning in a creek, a good twenty minutes' walk away. Louie of course was there before us all, but we made our way, single file through the forest.

Though I was last in line, somehow I managed to get stung by the infamous stinging tree. The small needle-like fibres from the tree are like a hollow glass tube that allows a toxin to be inserted into the skin. A bit like having nerve pain from a broken tooth. It managed to brush me right between the legs from my knees to my upper thigh. The men said we needed to turn back because there was no way I could work, especially in water, as it was well known to intensify the pain tenfold. I refused and said I would work anyway. They reluctantly agreed to continue on our way. The truth was when I first got into the water, it was excruciating. But the water was so cold that I believe it contracted my skin and pushed out the fibres. Usually, a sting from this tree can hurt for hours, or in some cases years, but I was able to work and woke up the next morning with no lasting effect.

On the day we packed to leave, Louie presented me with a container of gold. I could not believe my eyes. I did not know that we had indeed found any gold at all let alone that I would be paid in gold. It seemed also to be way too much gold or payment for a young boy like me. He assured me I had earnt it and thanked me like I was a man. I felt proud and worthy. I had no clue of the gold's worth but did feel rich. It turned out to be about an ounce and a half, equivalent to around four to five hundred dollars in those days. That was way more than what I had ever earned before.

Cross-Dressing & Croc Surfing

Still looking for a real job, I landed a beauty. It was as a landscape gardener at the Moon River Resort in Trinity Park. These days it is an affluent marina estate but back then it was only really a caravan park with a fancy name. But my boss was none other than the great Norm Provan. Norm had been the captain and coach of the Australian Rugby League Team. He was 6 feet 4 inches and seemed to be 3 feet across the shoulders. In his mid-fifties, his hands were twice the size of mine. Although I used all my effort, Norm could easily do double the amount of work that I could.

Living at the next beach, it only took a ten-minute walk to get to work each morning even though there was a small creek for me to cross on the way. My other alternative was to ride my noisy two-stroke dirt motorbike through the private cane fields or along the main road without a licence or registration. The creek bed was sand, and I knew it well. On the way to work one day, it had been raining, and I noticed the tide was unusually high and the water very murky. Because it was stinger season, when painful jellyfish were abundant and whose tentacles had been known to send people into cardiac arrest, I wore the commonly used garment for such a creek crossing: women's stockings.

My custom was to carry my shoes and lunch above my head with one hand while I used the other to steady myself against the tide. As I entered the water this day, the current was very strong, flowing the fastest on the surface, incoming from the sea. The water got deeper and deeper. Soon I found it up to my chin. I began to tread water. Just then, my foot landed on a surface that seemed to lift me up at least a foot. It then lifted me again as it moved. I knew it was something alive and I wasn't hanging around to find out what it was. I lifted both my legs like a gazelle and made like one of those mosquitos that skirt along the water's surface. The tide took me downstream and back to the same side that I had started on, only this time into the mangroves where I knew there were crocodiles for sure. I managed to make my way through the knee-high mud and decided to stay home that day. My mates stir me about the 'live log' and the 'quick turtle' but it was enough for me to risk the motorbike ride from then on, at least most of the time.

Strangulation by Uncertain Burton

I continued to explore the tropical paradise where I was now living. There were great rivers and mighty waterfalls. The fishing was awesome. The rainforest had the smell of new growth and was an adventure playground with a myriad of bird songs and the movement of abundant wildlife.

The hills and streams had gold, and the ground sprouted crystals. At the age of eighteen, I lived on the picturesque Ellis Beach for months with a bunch of wild characters, mostly naked, while we ate from the surrounding mangoes, bananas, lychees and coconuts. These people's lifestyle and wisdom of nature diminished any shame and embarrassment I had of nakedness. They managed to unveil and dismantle any of my city logic. I had also saved enough money from my welfare payments to buy a car and eventually settled on the Tablelands above Cairns in a little town called Kuranda.

A friend of mine suggested that we get away for a while camping and fishing. I had first met Drake in a social card game circle called Oh Hell. He suggested that we go to Cedar Bay, a remote beach between Bloomfield and Cooktown. Drake was about twenty years my senior and a veteran of living in the bush. Up for adventure, I agreed, so we packed our gear and set off in his old Ford sedan. We drove north and crossed the Daintree River via the ferry. Just past Cape Tribulation, we came across the famous Daintree Blockade. The year was 1984 and a large contingent of protesters were camping in the area and had been there for almost a year. They had attracted international media attention, promoting the conservation of the pristine forest to the north and protesting against the proposed permanent road the government intended to build.

There was a track, though only the game driver would attempt it, with slippery slopes and perilous potholes dotted all the way to Cooktown. We were seasoned and thought we would give it a go. And while we were both conservation-minded and believed in sustainability, we knew a road was inevitable and needed for the many communities north. We stayed for a while and enjoyed the diverse philosophies, including that of the Church of the Holy Molecule, one of a few strange movements within the protest community. People were dug into the ground with only their heads poking out, some were camped in trees and others chained themselves to trees.

Eventually, the original rough dirt track was replaced with a permanent wider one, only better because it was more regularly maintained. When it was finally completed, we were amongst the first to attempt to drive it, along with some of the hippies and greenies that had protested so long.

About two-thirds of the way there, we stopped the car in readiness to cross the beautiful Bloomfield River. The crossing was not that far from the mouth of the river that met the sea. As such, in those parts, it was crocodile-infested. Luckily for us, the current was strong, and the water was clear and shallow in that area. Even so, the river was tidal and warranted an inspection before crossing. The riverbed was rocky, and it was well known that it was better to cross on the side where the rocks were smaller. We ventured into the water to about halfway across the river until we were satisfied that we knew which side to cross. We cautiously drove ahead and successfully navigated our way through.

Not far past the crossing, we passed the Wujal Wujal Christian 'Mission.' Across the entrance were big signs 'no white men' and 'no trespassers'; it was very intimidating. Soon we arrived at the private property of a friend, Doug, where we were to park our car while we took the day walk over the mountain and into the bay. We did the traditional bush call before getting too close to his house and gave a 'Cooee' out loud, to no response.

As we approached, we heard what seemed like a bit of moaning. Concerned, we rushed in to find Doug slumped on the floor. He had apparently been beaten and robbed. We stayed the night and tended to his injuries. The next morning, he seemed stable, thanked us, gave us some extra supplies and bid us well on our journey.

As we ascended the mountain range into Cedar Bay, I could see the appeal that it had. It was a long, half-moon-shaped beach, dotted with coconut palms and had various streams running from the mountains into the sea. It was totally secluded, only accessible by foot or by sea. With not a soul in sight, we set about making a camp on the beach. We enjoyed each other's company and skills for a few days but then decided to make separate camps and basked in the serenity.

I could see some decent sized fish in the streams and thought I would have a go at spearing one. Having found a straight sapling, I whittled away at it and sharpened one end. Attempt after attempt yielded nothing. Nearing the end of a whole day, I could not understand why I missed the fish every time. I decided to put my face in the water to look at what was going on. It was only then that I realised the fish were not in the same place when I looked at them from under the water as they were when I looked at them from above the water. The water refracted the light and changed the position of the fish according to its depth and size. It was as though I had become an enlightened caveman. I ate my first speared fish that night.

Drake and I did not see each other for a couple of days. When we crossed paths eventually, he shared with me some

coconut oil that had formed from a perfect mixture of the coconut cracking and allowing just enough air in, along with the
right amount of sun. We meandered along the beach together
and talked about our past couple of days. Apparently, Drake
had made friends with a coconut. He introduced it to me, and
being young and naïve, I was half expecting it to speak to me
as well. It did not.

Drake had no sooner crossed over a creek in front of me
when I noticed some movement in the bush just off the sand.
I looked up to see a very large boar. It had long tusks and
scruffy, wiry hair. As soon as it saw me, it grunted and charged
straight towards me. All I could think of to do was to run. I
yelled out to Drake, 'Pig!'

He saw me running straight along the beach but knew that
I could not outrun it. He yelled back, 'Swim out to sea, they
can't swim,' and I immediately took his advice. When I was in
deep water, I looked back. The pig was walking away, and
Drake was up a tree.

That night the brightest full moon came up from behind a
perfectly still sea. Its brilliance lit up the beach as though it
was an overcast day. We were drawn to the ocean and waded
out into the water. The tide was low, and we could walk out
for a great distance. We were excited to see lots of large fish,
swimming slowly, apparently mesmerised by the moon. We
decided to do some spearing and caught as many as we knew
we could eat.

Our adventure finally ended when we realised we had to
head back to sign our dole forms for our welfare payment.

The trip south was far from smooth. We thanked Doug for allowing us to park our car on his property, had a couple of rums, filled our stomachs and felt good to go. We pulled up at the Bloomfield River, and I undid the seatbelt to get out and check the depth. Without warning, Drake put his foot down and started to speed across the river.

I yelled at him, 'What are you doing? You should let me check the depth!'

He yelled back, 'Shut up! It's hard enough driving on these rocks as it is!'

I yelled again, 'But you're on the wrong side!'

With that, there was a huge bang and we came to a screeching halt. We had hit a large rock.

The water was just below the door level, so I thought that I could probably dive underneath to dislodge the rock. I tried a few times, but the rock was too big, and I only succeeded in burning myself on the exhaust pipe. Drake suggested that I jump up and down on the boot while he accelerated back and forth. It did not work. Then he suggested that I try jumping up and down on the bonnet, while he did the same. The only thing those things did was dent the car. After about half an hour of trying different things, the tide was rising and the sun was going down. We were entering … the crocodile zone.

We finally decided we had to bail and grabbed as much gear as we could before heading to the other side of the river. Setting up camp for the night, we decided to light a big fire to keep away the crocodiles. In the middle of the night, I needed to take a leak. I looked around the campsite with the torch and to the immediate area of the river to make sure it was safe.

I decided for some reason to shine the torch in the direction of the car. To my horror, it was gone. I thought to myself that the tide must have risen so high and become strong enough to take the car down the stream. I dreaded telling Drake in the morning.

At first light, I heard Drake stir and thought I would break it to him gently, so as not to make him too upset. He moaned but seemed to take it well. He crawled from the tent and stood up to stretch. Suddenly, he swiftly dived back into the tent and thrust his hands around my neck. He squeezed and yelled, 'You little mongrel, why would you lie? Your city ways drive me crazy and now you try to mess with me?'

Choking and confused, I tried to make sense of what he was saying. I felt my eyes bulging and the veins in my forehead pulsating. He shook me and squeezed me tighter. I realised that the car had not been taken down the river but simply the water had risen over the roof and now that the tide had dropped, the car was visible again. I managed to mutter my thoughts. Drake realised what had happened and let me go.

We made a cup of tea and contemplated our options. Knowing that the river was still salty being so close to the sea, we believed that because the car had been submerged, the electrics would be shot and there was little chance we would ever get the car started again. Nevertheless, we could not just leave the car in the middle of the river.

As we sat, ever aware of any sudden movement from the water, we heard a vehicle. A four-wheel drive approached and stopped when it saw our car. They offered to tow it out for us. We broke their rope and thanked them for their attempt. Another four-wheel-drive also broke their rope trying to help us. A third four-wheel-drive had a chain. It broke. They suggested we go to Wujal Wujal because they had a bulldozer. Drake and I looked at each other wide-eyed and gulped.

We made a short and long stick. We drew, and Drake got the short draw. Our plan was to offer them some money or a six-pack of beer. If I had not heard from Drake within an hour, I was to come looking for him. We shook hands as though we might never see each other again.

Though I had no watch, it seemed it had been more than an hour. I prepared myself for the worst, which in my mind involved being speared, then set off after him. I was only about halfway across the river when I heard the low rumble of heavy machinery. Around the corner, a bulldozer appeared with Drake hanging off the side. With some wrangling, he had managed to secure the help of the bulldozer but only with a full carton of beer. The bulldozer had no trouble pulling the car out and the driver waved us goodbye like we were true idiots.

Of course, the car would not start, so we made the decision to carry what we could on our back and stash the rest of our belongings in the bush to collect another day. We were just about ready to start walking when I heard a motorbike was crossing the river. I stood up to see the rider fall off the bike about halfway across. I immediately began to run to his aid. He saw me and yelled out, 'Don't worry, mate, sometimes I drop my motorbike three times a day in this river!'

I stopped running, and he jumped back on and rode away in seemingly one swift motion. When he reached our side, he stopped and thanked me for attempting to help him. He could see us with our backpacks on, standing next to our car, and asked us what we were doing. We explained what had happened. He said that his brothers were mechanics and were following him not far behind in a four-wheel drive. They would be there in a few minutes and could surely get our car going again. We were humbled by his gesture but honestly did not believe the car would start again.

As the mechanics examined the car, they declared that because the petrol cap had held fast and no water had entered the fuel, it was entirely possible to have the car going again within a couple of hours. They removed the spark plugs and the shaft below the distributor cap. Putting the car in gear, they towed it so that the water spewed out of the holes where the spark plugs had been. We waited for a while for things to dry out and then put everything back together. To our amazement, the car started. We gifted them a large handful of dope and drove away very thankful.

No sooner had we left the area before we got stuck in the next creek. We did not know whether to laugh or cry. We were only there a few minutes when another four-wheel-drive approached. They seemed to be some sort of government employees and were very disgruntled at the thought of having to help us out as they could not get around us. They grunted that we should not drive such a crappy vehicle under the conditions but towed us out of their way and left in a huff.

We approached the last steep climb at the bottom of a mountain, just before Cape Tribulation. As Drake and I rounded a corner that had a long drop-off to one side and a steep mountain going up on the other, we could see a long, dangerous-looking straight climbing upwards before us. The car seemed unsafe as we ascended slowly up the single lane of dirt, while we watched the ground over one side of the mountain disappear far below.

About two-thirds of the way to the top, it began to sprinkle with rain. The car crawled for a little further up the mountain, when the unthinkable happened. Our wheels began to spin. If we were to put on the brakes, we would slide backwards and most likely over the steep side. If we tried to reverse backwards, it was unlikely that we could turn quickly enough without sliding at the sharp bottom corner and thus going over the edge.

The stark reality was that our lives were at stake. If we were to jump out of the car, hopefully we could get clear of it and not be run over, though the side Drake was on had the steep drop-off. Either way, we would lose the car. We could not go forwards. We could not go backwards. Attempting to stop, the car would begin to slide. We sat there with the wheels spinning, but the car was beginning to slide backwards. All of this happened within seconds.

Drake yelled for me to get out and try to wedge a rock under a wheel. I imagined the wheel spitting the rock out into my face. I then imagined the car simply rolling back over the rock and the car squashing me. It was either that I attempted to do it, or we lose the car or maybe our lives. I dived out and to my amazement found a decent size rock right next to me. I yelled out that I had found one.

Drake yelled back, 'Do it when I hit the brakes!'

I picked up the rock and positioned myself to the side of the car. 'Now!' I shoved the rock in place. The car rolled over it. I was disappointed but not surprised. I turned around and looked again, seeing a much bigger rock.

I yelled out, 'Let's try again!' and picked it up with all my strength. He hit the brakes. The car stopped.

Drake took no chances and jumped from the car. We sat down silently, except for the heavy breathing. After we regained our composure, we discussed the fact that we may be there for quite a while, waiting for the next vehicle to possibly tow us to the top of the hill. We were right. Not another single vehicle came all day.

When dusk approached, we decided that we should set up a camp for the night. Unfortunately, there was no space in the bush, and everything was on a steep angle anyway. We tried to pitch our tent on the road itself. It looked ridiculous on such a slant and was very impractical. We attempted to sleep and in the middle of the night were awoken by the sound of a vehicle. Luckily for us, it had approached from the top of the hill. The driver said there would be no problem in towing us up the mountain. He hooked us up with his winch, and we made it safely to the top. On arriving back in Kuranda, Drake dropped me off and left the car at the rubbish tip.

Inmates of the Lost World

It was 1987, and at age nineteen, while staying with my sister on Black Mountain Road in Kuranda, I came to know some very unusual locals. This intriguing bunch would pass by our door every so often on their way to and from a hippie commune deep within the rainforest. They invited me to their secret location one time, and being inquisitive, I was happy to follow. The narrow winding track went up and down hills, over creeks and two kilometres later into a small clearing with a few scattered buildings. I was told the property was owned by a mad psychiatrist who had once lived there but now was happy to allow any nature-loving, wild-looking individual to live there. The main building had all the structural beams but very few walls. Vines replaced some walls and any furniture had the true shanty look. Naked and half-naked people could be seen doing some gardening while others enjoyed a smoke and a cuppa.

I found myself drawn to what I now know was referred to as Inmates, or The Lost World. As I visited more regularly, I eventually found my place and took up permanent residence. There were competitions to see who could live on mangoes the longest and what was the highest tree one was willing to jump out of, in order to scare the other, on their morning walk to wash in the creek. The uncrowned king of the hippies was undoubtedly Corey the Banana Man. His skin seemed to be so soft yet he would often ask me to punch him in the stomach as hard as I could, to prove that he would not flinch, but that his stomach wobbled just like rubber.

After many months of living with nature and amongst the array of strange people, there was a particularly unruly man that I spied randomly chopping down vegetation, including the prized vines that made our walls. I arced up and chased him from the property telling him to never return. That same day, I returned with an extremely beautiful girl that I had met on my walk to town. It was evident that these acts had handed me the new crown as King of the Inmates of the Lost World.

Mafia Thriller Stripper

Around six months later, after deciding to join civilisation again, I ventured into the town of Kuranda. I had in mind that I would look for a job but expected no offers, wearing no underpants and the see-through sarong that was my usual look. Just then, a girl I knew asked me if I wanted a job dancing from Cairns to the Gold Coast. She told me I would be paid $100 a night with all transport and accommodation included. Without thinking, I said yes. She asked me to be at the Edgehill Community Hall for choreography at 9 a.m. Monday morning.

I arrived first, followed by around twenty extremely gorgeous girls. My excitement could almost not be contained when the last girl arrived, and I realised I was the only male. The choreographer had us all do a session of aerobics first up. The girls giggled at me because I struggled to keep pace. I was asked by the choreographer to sort through a bag of clothes and accessories and choose some to take off as I danced to my choice of music. I hesitated at first, but then looked around to remember it was all girls and I was actually in my glory.

The choreographer nonchalantly informed us that the owners of the 'Night Clubs' did not require us to take off all of our clothes, but they would like it. It finally clicked. I was a stripper!

Trying to contain my excitement, I stayed in the flow of the moment, choosing the song 'Thriller' to strip to. I had begun to get right into the tease when a man walked in. I became immobilised. He approached the choreographer with an angry demeanour and left after just a few words. The choreographer announced that it was the end of the session for the day and when we would meet again. Before I left, she called me aside. She told me that the boss wanted to meet me and where and when to do it. A grave disappointment came over me coupled with alarm. I knew the place she wanted me to go. I also knew that he was local mafia. I visualised the meeting and how by them offering me a job, I would now 'owe' them. I also foresaw my future as his 'boy.' I made the painstaking decision not to meet him and forego my dream trip of travelling with a bus full of stripper girls.

Jive Dude Turkey

The First Nations peoples of Kuranda were a friendly and happy lot. The beautiful rainforest that surrounded them would surely make anybody happy. Most people in Kuranda seemed to be stoners, and everybody said they were an artist. I took jobs from landscaping and beekeeping to warden of the hostel, rainforest tour guide and laboratory assistant. Having volunteered for a number of years at the community amphitheatre, I helped to build structures and take care of visiting bands. I also regularly helped my friend, 'Major StarGazer' with his community radio show, and my on-air name was 'Jive Dude Turkey Paul'. Joining the local theatre gave me an exciting challenge, and it was a great thrill when I began to perform live. It was captivating watching people I knew suddenly transform and rehearse in vivid dramatic expression. My adrenaline always pumped when I knew anyone was watching me. It seemed my ego as a young man was insatiable. Eventually, I worked my way to payment as a professional actor.

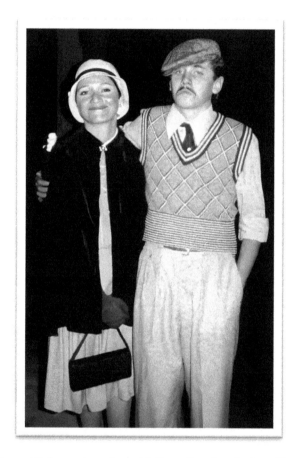

Bonnie and I dressed up for a 1940s radio play. I played both the criminal and the policeman.

Deb had broken up with Phil about six months ago and seemed a little sad to me. I had been thinking of a way to cheer her up when I decided to visit the Kuranda Amphitheatre.

It was a typical day with rehearsals for plays, community workshops and preparations for concerts, along with general maintenance of the grounds. Everybody there was a volunteer and constant laughter could be heard. Late in the afternoon, I was attracted to a group of people conversing loudly. I overheard a man that I had seen before, but didn't know personally, commenting that he was going out on the town that night 'raging'. I interrupted and asked him if he would mind taking my sister out. He looked at me wide-eyed and said, 'I know your sister, sure I'll take her out, but you have to come and ask her with me.' *What a big wuss*, I thought, but I agreed.

On arrival at Debbie's place, a little cottage in the rainforest on Black Mountain Road, I announced, 'Deb, I'm minding Holly tonight (who was about five years old), and Barry is taking you out.'

She said, 'Who's Barry?' to which Barry, who was behind me, said in a very Pommy accent, 'I'm Barry.'

When their eyes met it was as though she melted like a little puppy dog.

It seemed things must have gone well because within about a year, in early 1988, I got word that my sister was pregnant to Barry. I was in the outback at the time and a friend of mine, Chris, was working for me as a carpenter. We came back to town to arrive a day after the birth. As we approached the hospital bed, because it was Christmas time, Santa Claus arrived as well. We gave gifts of frankincense, jewels and potpourri, and in the basket of potpourri flowers, I placed a crystal star.

A couple of weeks later we had heard that they had named the baby. I tracked Debbie down to the Kuranda Amphitheatre where a music festival was happening. As I entered the gates, Greg, a friend of mine, handed me a crystal star and said, 'Here brother, here's a key to your heart.'

I approached my sister and asked her what she had named the baby. To my amazement, the child had been named Crystal-Star. Debbie had picked Crystal and Barry had chosen Star, so they made it into one name. I showed her what Greg had just given me and called him over. They didn't even know each other. I asked her if she had named the baby because of the crystal star I had given her, but she said, 'What crystal star?'

She hadn't even seen it; apparently, it had fallen down through the flowers of the potpourri. I was amazed at the seeming coincidence.

My Gypsie

I loved going to the local markets to try new fruits, socialise and enjoy the variety of eccentric buskers. One day a very beautiful girl caught my eye. Just then, a gust of wind blew up her skirt while she modestly attempted to hold it down. When she looked up and saw me looking at her, she let it go a couple of times. I nearly fainted. Some friends knew her and told me her name was Gypsie.

Soon after, I saw Gypsie again at the Kuranda Amphitheatre. It was my 18th birthday, and I was having a celebration. Gypsie had been invited by a friend of mine and was preparing food in the kitchen. I pretended not to notice her and started faking a laugh with my friends. In those days I was known by the name of Hippie Paul.

Gypsie then approached me and said, 'Aren't you Happy Paul?'

I decided that I was indeed Happy Paul. Looking into her eyes, the rest of the world melted away. Never had I seen or spoken to a girl more captivating. She was sweet and intelligent, and looked at life differently than anybody I had ever met. I wasted no time in pursuing her. We flirted and played like children. For some mysterious reason, the gods favoured me and Gypsie became my girlfriend.

Gypsie grew up in the rainforest of Cape Tribulation, where she lived a very natural existence, mostly naked. She had never eaten meat, drank alcohol, smoked cigarettes or eaten junk food in her life. She was always helping people who were down on their luck. Gypsie and I loved nature and would spend a lot of time on the beach. She loved making necklaces from flowers and cracking open coconuts with whatever was close. I remember how she showed me to suck honey from a bunch of Lantana flowers, then to throw them in the air so that they would gently arrange themselves amongst our hair. She looked like a fairy angel.

Sometimes I would give her things I thought she would cherish, only to see somebody else with whatever it was soon after. She had no attachment to material possessions. It wasn't until later in my life that I truly experienced the power and freedom of not being attached to physical things.

Gypsie would find a way to use everything that we had seemingly more than once. She always said, 'We can afford everything but waste.' In the heart of Gypsie, deep in her spirit, was the ability to make people see their flaws and nakedness without embarrassing them. If she saw people eating junk

48

food constantly, she sometimes said, 'A baby knows the chocolate it's eating is worth it but what it doesn't know is that its teeth are worth much more.'

By far the best job I ever had was when working on a property just about ten miles out of town. I worked for a great man named Geoff. He was a natural therapist and property developer. Geoff only had one leg but could still do twice the amount of work that I could. I was his carer, building project assistant and residential landscape gardener. Gypsie lived there with us too. On the property, there were a couple of beautiful white horses - Spanish dancing Andalusians. I rode them by their mane, bareback and sometimes bare everything, when I came out naked and caught them eating from the herb garden first thing in the morning. The property was nine acres of trees, plants and gardens. I had helped build waterfalls through the house, took care of his horses and nurseries, and had done various landscaping jobs.

A knock on the door one day turned out to be a young couple – Mick, Valerie and their daughter Gigi, asking if we knew of a good creek in the area to camp at. I asked Geoff for his recommendation. He told them that they were welcome to camp on his land. The new family were so lovely that they were invited to stay permanently. Mick, a carpenter, was allowed to build a house there for the family.

Gypsie had a way of making everybody that she knew feel special. Every time that Gypsie introduced me to somebody new, she always said that they were her best friend. Walking through the markets with Gypsie was like having a movie star to protect. People would want to talk to her and ask her to come to anything that was happening. She once told me, 'Being happy is living. Living is praying. Praying is praising and when you're praising, you're happy. Life's a beautiful cycle like that.'

I loved her more than life itself.

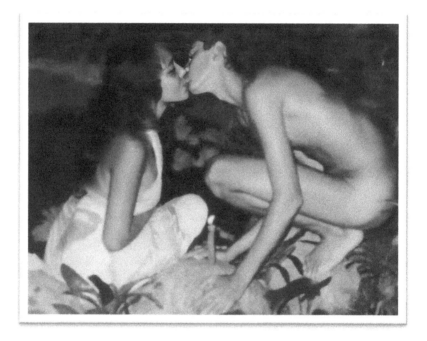

Kissing Gypsie over some of my landscaping.

The Beaming Preacher

Ellinjaa Falls was in a luscious area of the Tablelands. Friends of mine had named their new baby girl and had invited me to a celebration of her birth near the falls. The area is truly the wet tropics with meandering fogs and mists rolling over the mountains and through the valleys.

I stayed at the party for a few hours enjoying the good company and magical scenery before I decided to begin the two-hour drive back to Kuranda. I was about to leave when someone asked me if I was hungry and wanted some soup. I had said yes before they told me of the magic mushrooms in the soup. I had tried magic mushrooms once before, but they seemed to have no effect on me. I had the soup, believing I would most likely once again not be affected.

I began to say my goodbyes when the host asked me a question. 'Brother, I know that you did not bring these kids, but since you are going back to Kuranda, do you mind taking that bunch of kids over there with you?'

I told him that I could surely do that as I turned to see who he was talking about. I looked in amazement at this bunch. Every single one of them I did not like for one reason or another. There was one that I knew had been accused of assault, one had robbed the local store, another that was the town bully and another I had suspected of stealing my sister's handbag.

At twenty, I was two or three years older than them and though two of them were bigger than me, I relished in the thought of rounding them up and began to plot a lesson.

Having delivered them the news of their fate, we all jumped in my van and began our journey. No sooner had I started the engine when I felt the mushrooms take effect. My eyes seemed to grow large. I had an acute awareness of every sound. I appeared to be able to see in the darkness ahead, as though a floodlight was before me. I didn't realise at first that I had begun to drive without the headlights on but then decided to keep them off as I felt confident that I could see perfectly and it would give me more impact for my upcoming sermon.

A great peace came over me as I smirked while absorbing my passengers' complaints. I calmly announced that everybody would remain silent as I spoke about ethics and principles. The road seemed clearer as the van gathered speed. We were now doing 100 km/hour along the highway in the middle of the night, with no headlights. The journey included mountain ranges with precarious turns and deep drop-offs to the side.

I raised my voice as I talked about respect for people, places and things. I preached about lying and stealing, aggression and integrity as my passengers begged for headlights, to be let out of the vehicle and for their life. When I said something that I believed had hit home, I paused with long silences. I think that over those two hours, my passengers truly believed they were going to die, and my words would be the last that they would hear.

When we arrived in Kuranda, I was surprised to see how calmly they exited the van, a single file of mute zombies. They walked away slowly in different directions, and I never heard about them again.

Having felt justified back then in believing I may have curbed them from their behaviours spiralling further into detriment, I realise now that I could have caused significant long-term psychological damage to these young punks and these days would offer them a workshop that I have created called 'The Higher Desire', which will be included in my next book.

My Life Changes Forever

My family and I were quite close and kept in contact regularly. When my sister rang me one day, I could hear in her voice that she sounded distraught. She had dreamt that I'd dived into some water and couldn't move again. She begged me not to go swimming. As I was a fit 20-year-old man who loved the water, I would regularly swim every day or two. I found it hard, but for weeks, I resisted the urge to go swimming. I had at the time been helping my brother to restore an old Falcon, when seemingly out of instinct, we decided to pack everything up.

The next day was a particularly beautiful day. It was four days before Christmas, and I woke early and came across Valerie, the lady who had been invited to stay on the property with her partner, Mick, and their children. Because I had been working solidly on the days preceding, both on the car with my brother and around the property, she offered to give me a massage. I was very thankful.

Some months later she relayed something to me that I had said during the massage, words that were to echo loudly in the future: 'I just want to lie down and never have to get up again.'

Because it was such a lovely day, I decided to sneak out of the house just in case the boss wanted me to work that day. Geoff caught me about to drive away and asked me to do an errand for him in town. I had completely forgotten about what my sister had told me and it seemed like a perfect day for a swim. As I walked through the main street of Kuranda, expectedly, as I had done many times before, I happened upon a lady friend of mine, Rachel. It so happened that Rachel asked me if I would like to go for a swim. I told her I had an errand to do, and she said that I could pick her up along the way if I decided to go. I soon finished my business and decided I would indeed go for a swim.

Calling into my friend Jasper's house, I found Rachel there too. We all set off on our way for a swim and parked the car at the end of Weir Road as we headed towards the water of the weir along the railway track. Together we walked down the stairs and went and sat on 'our rock', as we had many times before. It was a wide-open space with the large rock slowly undulating over some ten metres or more. There were a number of high water marks from times when the river had flooded. The Barron River itself was always a muddy brown, and apparently, this was caused by the run-off from the many farms upstream, along with gushing tributaries from wet areas scattered across the Tablelands.

Jasper and Rachel began to chat, while I decided to go for a swim. I took off my shirt and waded into the water up to my knees. I assumed the weir was at its normal full capacity as it had been raining for the last few nights. I leaned forward and began to breaststroke, with my head just slightly under the surface of the water. I had only swum a few body lengths when my head hit a rock that wasn't usually there. It stunned me, and I felt a sharp pain across the top of my head. My natural instinct was to feel what had happened to the top of my head and to lift my face out of the water for a breath. I could not move my arms or my head and simply floated to the top of the water. I tried to squirm and roll over, but nothing happened. After a short time, I could not hold my breath any longer. I began to inhale water, and I watched the river turn red as I bled. My eyes began to close as I felt my consciousness drifting away. I called out to God to let me live.

In that moment, the freedom and vigour that I enjoyed as a happy young man with a healthy body was to be lost for the rest of my life.

Why the Channel 7 Chopper Chills Me to My Feet

I knew that I'd knocked my head, but I didn't know why I was paralysed from the neck down. I later found out that the water level had been dropped four feet by the authorities to create a waterfall for the tourist train to see. They hadn't informed the locals.

With no energy left to fight, my spirit was at peace with the resolve of leaving the body for the great beyond. Just then I was jolted back to life as Rachel spun me over, and I saw the light of the sky again. I managed to breathe as she pulled me over to the riverbank and cradled my head. We knew something serious had happened but did not understand what a spinal injury was. The sensation from my neck down was similar to that of hitting a funny bone. An intense tingling and at the same time, a burning sensation.

We decided it was best not to get me out of the water but instead to send Jasper to run for medical help. Soon our local doctor Ashley arrived, along with paramedics, police and onlookers. The doctor asked me if I had any pain, to which I said not really. He still gave me an injection that made me drowsy.

The then well-liked businessman Christopher Skase (now infamous) happened to have a helicopter passing by. He directed it to my rescue. It arrived soon after and as there were no flat areas for it to land, it hovered and struggled to balance straight, with one landing skid above the water and the other on the rock where the paramedics had gently placed me on a stretcher. As the paramedics were putting me into the helicopter, another helicopter from Channel 7 came onto the scene as it tried to film everything from above.

Suddenly a loud chopping noise was heard from the sky and as we looked up, we could see that the Channel 7 helicopter had clipped the top of the trees and was starting to come down sidewards towards us and the onlookers. People were screaming and running in different directions. The paramedics did look up for a moment, but then looked at each other, shook their heads, shrugged their shoulders and continued to carefully load me into the rescue helicopter.

The paramedics risked their lives to save me further injury. Their selfless act is something I will forever be grateful for. It is something that I have pondered many times in life, and it has ensured my appreciation of the true nature and compassion of humanity. The Channel 7 helicopter somehow managed to straighten up and hastily flew away.

I must have allowed the painkiller to do its job after that, as the next thing I remember was the distorted faces of friends in the Cairns Base Hospital. This was then followed by the awkward ride on a stretcher in the front section of a commercial airliner to the Spinal Injuries Unit of the Princess Alexandria Hospital in Brisbane. Further painkillers ensued before I was abruptly awoken by a man saying, 'Hit it harder, hit it harder with the hammer, nurse!' as I felt a blow to the side of my head.

I quickly tried to react as I could see about half a dozen people standing around me, one swinging a hammer at my head. They were frantic and injected me with yet another drug. I later learned that this was the hospital's way of putting traction into your skull, to hold you so that you don't move. The traction is two steel prongs piercing your skull, wounds that are maintained open, to stop the skin growing around them. There is eleven pounds of weight hanging off them from the top of your head so you can't move and injure your spine further.

Some four days later, I opened my eyes to the doctor saying, 'Happy Christmas.' My Christmas present was an orange juice that the doctor had to help me to drink. I was halfway through drinking it when he blurted, 'It's my professional duty to tell you that you'll probably never walk again.' Straight away I hit back, 'Who told you that, doc? Don't believe them, eh?'

He gasped and muttered, 'Gee, I wish everybody would say that to me so soon after an injury.'

I learned that I had fractured my spine and bruised my spinal cord around the third to fourth vertebrae from the top of my neck. There were few recoveries. At twenty years old, I would likely be a quadriplegic for the rest of my life.

I had no feeling from just above my nipples down. A burning sensation replaced all other feeling. I could just move my arms. I couldn't use my hands. I couldn't feel my willy. I had a lot of water on my lungs from inhaling it at the river, and the doctors were considering a tracheotomy to help me breathe. My parents were told I would die.

After spending a number of weeks in intensive care, my spirit prevailed. I was released to the general ward and began to regain some vitality. A benefit concert was organised for me in Kuranda, raising thousands of dollars to help me and my family through this traumatic time. Local bands performed and businesses donated goods to sell and auction. During the middle of the concert, I received a phone call at the hospital from the organisers, and they passed around the phone so that I could speak to people. Then they put me on a loudspeaker to speak to the crowd. I had just written a song, which they asked me to sing. The familiar and friendly voices in the phone call gave me the strength and incentive to try to regain any sense of a normal life.

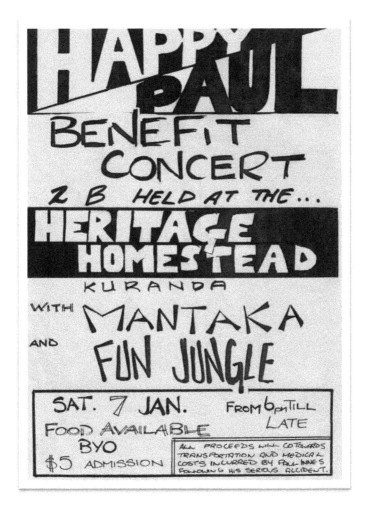

Announcing my benefit concert

My brother Danny, his partner Anne-Marie and their daughter April flew with me from Cairns when I first sustained the injury and tried to help me cope while they dealt with their own feelings from the trauma. My mum had moved back and forward from Cairns to Sydney and was now living in Sydney again. Though Mum and Dad were still separated, they travelled together from Sydney and arrived at the same time as the rest of my family. I was having all sorts of medication for various things to do with my injury. Over the next couple of weeks, I stabilised. I was kept fairly well drugged and had an injection every four hours for the pain in the back of my neck. I had tubes hanging out of me everywhere, including from my willy. I had to have suppositories and do a crap in bed. It was humiliating, and I was beginning to become depressed.

I asked the head doctor about a cure. He said that they were not interested in a cure, but in care. I hounded him and paid for his subscription to the International Spinal Research Foundation. The same hospital has now become the first in the world to discover that nasal cells can be turned into stem cells and used in the healing of spinal cord injuries when they are at an early stage.

The muscle spasm tablets that I was taking began to make me hallucinate, so I was cut back to the bare minimum. As time went on, more people visited me, including physiotherapists who came daily to move my limbs. Occupational therapists made devices to help me become more independent.

Most people do not really understand what a spinal injury is. People have commonly asked me if being paralysed feels like you have no body from the injury site down. The truth is that your spinal cord is like the electrical cord of an appliance. Your brain being the source of electricity, your spinal cord being the electrical cord, and your body being the appliance. When the electrical cord of an appliance is damaged, the appliance just doesn't work properly anymore. When I had my injury, it was like hitting the funny bone in my neck, but the buzzing sensation (which some people experience as burning and pain) doesn't ever go away. And when I try to move my foot for instance, there is an electrical impulse that I feel in that region but it is not enough to force the muscles to move. It does, however, provide me with a sense of spatial awareness of my limbs and therefore the sensation that I still have a body.

An old mate of mine sat patiently beside my bed for nine months after my injury. John King or Jack Fisher, as he liked to be called, and I had been friends for a few years by that point, even though he was sixty-six years old and I was twenty. He had taken me under his wing when I was sixteen and taught me bits and pieces of all manner of things from bush crafts to Latin.

He now read me the collection of books written by Carlos Castaneda, which gave me vivid visions and I am sure influenced the hallucinations I experienced through too much muscle spasm medication. On discussions with Jack, he suggested that I had every chance of winning a court case for my injury against the government. We wrote to a barrister who also agreed we had a great chance of winning such a case and initiated proceedings pro bono. We began what became a six-year saga.

Over the months, I got somewhat stronger physically, but I did feel trepidation about leaving the hospital or being functional in society again. Lights irritated me, so I covered my eyes with black material. When I first watched the television there was a movie that began to portray some slight violence, but it was enough to remind me of my vulnerability and I became very distraught. I was feeling intimidated and defenceless because I couldn't protect myself like I had been able to before. I wasn't the man I used to be.

Along came the day I was allowed to get in a wheelchair. I thought that just getting around in a wheelchair might somehow be different and I might feel freer. I attempted to push myself and realised I couldn't move a foot because I was so weak. Nevertheless, like the other three guys in my room and the other thirty or so in the Spinal Unit, everyone was tasked by all staff to push themselves to the gym every day. I reeled in pain and used all my strength to move a couple of inches every minute or two. The physiotherapists stood back and watched as it took an hour to get there. I thought, *What cold, hard bitches!* When I look back now, I realise it was the only way to get me strong again.

I remember going out of the hospital for the first time with my brother-in-law Barry. We went to a street where he left me in the middle of the footpath while he was in one of the shops. It was humiliating that I couldn't get into the shop because of the step. It was also chilling to feel that I was susceptible to anything happening to me out there and that I couldn't protect myself anymore. I was a humbled man, a scared man, who wanted to get back to the hospital, to the security of sterility, the quietness of the wards, where there was empathy from the nurses and love from my family and friends. Where there also was some comfort from all the devices that had been designed for injuries such as mine. I felt that it was in that sanctuary I was able to find some peace, some relief.

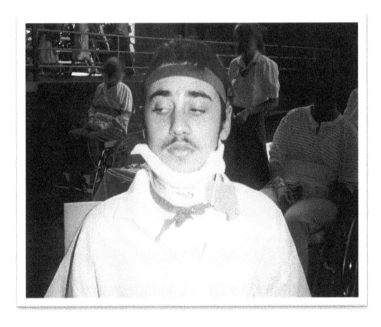

My first wheelchair race. They were gaining on me (not really).

As the months went by, I began to gain more self-confidence. The Guinness Book of World Records people came to visit the Spinal Unit to see if they could inspire any of the people that were stuck in bed for months to have a go at breaking some records. They asked if anyone wanted to have a go at the record for eating an apple suspended on a string in the least number of bites and the least number of minutes.

A young man named Tommy and I decided to have a go. We were not allowed to use our hands and had to have somebody else hold the string while we attempted to bite at the apple. According to the rules, you were allowed to have the person holding the string to swing the apple at you. Because an apple is fairly round, it's hard to sink your teeth into, so I asked the person who was holding mine to swing it at me. That just resulted in it smashing me in the mouth.

Eventually, I got it and had to eat every skerrick including the core, which was also the rule. We both were able to beat the record with four bites in eight minutes. My ego was too big, so I decided to have another go. I had taken two bites and time was running out. The only way to beat the record was to eat the rest of the apple in one bite. With an almighty lunge and a stretching of the lips, I did it! They also asked if anybody was willing to try to suck up water at the most straw lengths. Because I could do circular breathing on a digeridoo, I assumed reversing this would work. I had a go and was able to break the record with seventeen straw lengths. As the editor of the Spinal Injury Unit newsletter for the month, I wrote 'Paul Innes broke the record for having the biggest mouth and being the biggest sucker!'

My Angel Flies Free

My family rented a place nearby the hospital and visited every day. Gypsie would bring me juices and healthy food. After about six months, some ads appeared on television about an upcoming documentary featuring Gypsie and her family. It portrayed the idyllic existence she had growing up at Emmagen Creek. It showed their wild food diet and their naked lifestyle.

Because I could have been in rehabilitation for up to eighteen months, Gypsie and I agreed that it was time for her to go home, at least for a while. We kept in close contact. A couple of weeks later the documentary aired, and Gypsie became a bit of a national sensation. She was talked about in the hospital, newspaper, on radio and on television.

A few weeks passed, and I sat in bed reading a book. The man in the bed next to me watched his television. Suddenly, there was a news flash.

Gypsie had died.

She had committed suicide.

What was I hearing? *No, it is impossible,* I thought. It's some kind of mistake. She has run off to the bush and somehow faked her death.

As I tried to face what may have been the grim reality, I became distraught with emotion. Distress, anger, heartache, grief. My beloved, my world, my life.

I sank. I could not hear. There was a deafening silence. Everything went grey-green. I was numb.

Gypsie had been so sad and I never knew. She had only ever shared her love. Her love of the earth and nature, her path of harmlessness. Now she was gone, and the world had lost an inspiring hero.

Gypsie wrote me a letter a couple of weeks before I had my injury. Here is an excerpt from that letter:

All I really need is food, shelter and clothing. Not even that: if you're really wild U don't get cold. All I really need is the sun and the rain, which are in a pawpaw.

I've got so much love, I could be a breatharian.

I can't share all of me 'cause I've got to save some of me 4 me, that's my share. If everyone else gets and I miss out, I don't call that selfish – I call that unfair. Don't U? U know me. I like 2 make sure everyone gets their fair share and it's unfair if there's 5 people, 5 pieces of pawpaw, and 1 misses out because 1 person gets 2 pieces. If I don't look after myself as well, I'm being selfish 'cause I can't help the rest of the world from drowning if I'm drowning myself. If some 1 else has a hang-up should it be my hang-up 2? Or should I do my best to help (please) them without hurting myself? I don't have lust for any type of flesh. I don't make love, I give it.

Some people have sugar, some people have sex, even eat meat.

Some people don't have sugar in their tea because...

Some people don't drink tea, I never do. But everyone 2 their own thing, I reckon. Some people might prefer an orange rather than a cup of tea. Well, I say let them be if they'd rather have an orange and be healthy and live. Don't try and push sugar on them if they don't wish it.

Anyway, I'd die 4 you. I'd die 4 the whole world if God wanted me 2.

Gypsie made me a warrior.

I had been in hospital for eight months when Gypsie took her life. When I awoke the next morning, all the staff from the Spinal Unit were gathered around my bed to support me. They told me they could arrange for me to go home for the funeral. I went home but never came back.

The cathedral echoed with crying as Gypsie arrived in a white coffin. A number of streets surrounding had to be blocked off to allow the masses of people that mourned Gypsie Rebel.

All these years later, I have never forgotten about the special way that Gypsie looked at life, and the things she taught me. I only hope that I could be half the person that was my Gypsie.

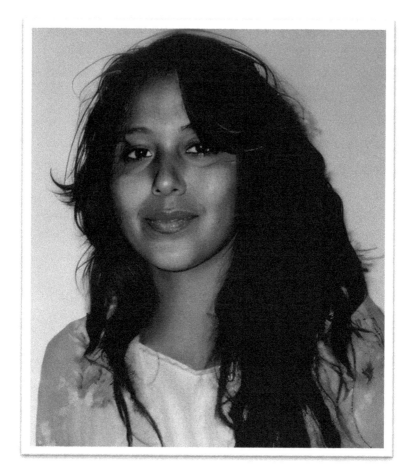

Gypsie Rebel.

Medication or Meditation?

My family soon whisked me away to a large open property on the Tablelands, where we stayed with my sister. They nurtured me and comforted me in a selfless, healing way. Friends came into my life to become carers; carers came into my life to become friends.

The community offered help in many ways. People would bring food and meals, offer to take me out and mow my lawn. The government offered to pay for carers and for medical supplies. The support was overwhelming and though it was hard to accept that I needed help, it was welcome.

As the months passed, my family regrouped and I moved into a house with my mum, my brother and his partner and child. As time went on, I learned what medication, medical equipment and supplies best suited my needs. It seemed that things changed endlessly and there was always something that had to be adjusted, repaired or trialled. The system had gaps and at times I found myself very frustrated. Along with my sister, my family took care of me 24/7 and sacrificed years of their own lives for my recovery to relative independence. Finally, at around age twenty-three, I was able to live by myself again albeit having the need for carers and a wheelchair to get around. I thank them sincerely and will be forever grateful. I am humbled by their devotion in my time of great need.

I became inspired and began to regain some self-worth. I decided to visit random old folks in nursing homes every Sunday. After a couple of years, it prompted me to start a service doing maintenance and gardening for people with disabilities and the aged in their own homes, utilising and supervising halfway-house prisoners and people doing community service.

Some hard cases tried to break me, but I always eventually broke them. I remember one burly bald-headed hallway-house prisoner tried to get out of mowing an old lady's lawn one day. Because I understood his culture and that they were mostly God-fearing, I promptly informed him that God was punishing me for being a sinner by confining me to this wheelchair and that he better not cross me otherwise he would be back in jail.

The government eventually adopted the idea and had me work for them from their office before turning it into a permanent program.

***

At some stage before my injury, I had a spiritual experience involving Jesus. Now that I was drifting in and out of church again, I eventually came to realise that there was no one God sitting on a sterilised throne in some antiseptic corner of the universe. I acknowledged that existence itself and the vastness of the cosmos was simply too profound and diverse for religion to interpret.

After my injury, my focus became more health and healing orientated, and I endured some intense self-directed therapies, which yielded slight improvements. I attended a workshop called Body Electronics, where people were learning to experience amazing healings. Many local alternative practitioners were attending. The workshop was held by Dr John Whittman Ray. This amazing man was a professor, medical doctor, chiropractor, naturopath and had degrees in chemistry, mathematics and physics. He had worked with Dr Bernard Jenson, the founder of iridology, studied with Hawaiian Kahuna witchdoctors and was also a lover of Jesus, Saint Germain and Sai Baba. All very cool in my books. Dr Ray taught alongside his wife and advocated that the practice of his teachings be done free of charge. The information he relayed to the people in the workshops inspired even the longest-serving practitioners.

The basis of his teachings centred on allowing an environment for spiritual, emotional, mental and physical healing. We were taught to apply these principles in a supportive group, through spiritual disciplines, emotional transmutations and mental focus. We also applied and received sustained acupressure, used natural supplements and transitioned to a raw food diet. For some people, it was a slow process, but for others with a strong constitution and metabolism, it was somewhat easy.

We were taught that fears are stop-signs in our growth and may even cause more fears to grow, yet we have the ability to re-experience, reinterpret and release ourselves by transmuting the old programming, while accessing and clearing the memory with our new understanding. We can do this with the power of forgiveness and loving appreciation because it gives us the opportunity to learn something new. This allows us to experience each moment as significant to our personal growth.

We also learned that we digest food at around 37 degrees, above which enzymes are killed. By cooking food, we must not only use the enzymes from our stomach but also from our skin, wrinkling us; our bones, weakening us; and our hair, greying us. These are the things that age us. If we put dead food in, we get death out of it.

I continued with the course for over a year and a half. I saw many amazing things happen. Some people with grey hair had it turn back to its original colour. Scars disappeared. Implanted metal rods that were seen on X-rays were now somehow re-placed by bone.

A particular couple who happened to be homosexual gave an astounding testimony during one certain session. They had originally joined the group because one came to heal his tennis elbow and the other his repetitive strain injury of the wrist. They announced that through the extreme discipline of the program, and particularly diet, it had balanced the chemicals in their body and in turn, their hormones. They told a stunned audience that they were both no longer attracted to males and were now attracted again to females. A burst of laughter spread throughout the room because people thought it was a joke. The two men stayed stone-faced and everyone realised they were serious. That's when many started to cry.

I know that some people are born with homosexual tendencies or have differences with such things as being born with an extra chromosome. I also now know that our diet can change the chemicals in our bodies. I have never been and will never be homophobic.

With the acupressure, we understood that there was a sequence of pulsations experienced in the fingertips when giving a person sustained acupressure during a healing session. We were only permitted to stop the session during certain sequences; otherwise, a person may have been worse off. During a particular theory session one day, we were told of a healing during Body Electronics that involved an exorcism. Dr Ray went on to explain in detail the events that led up to, and what happened during the exorcism. People in the audience confirmed they had been there during that session. We then began our usual practice where a person receives sustained-acupressure healing by up to six other people, when we were confronted with the same situation.

As was our usual routine after we'd our theory presented, we began our acupressure practice for the day. I was one of about six people chosen to be the recipient of the acupressure. Most times, there were between four to six people performing the acupressure on the recipient.

I was about ten feet away from the next table where a well-known local naturopath, Lillian, was on another massage table receiving acupressure. About half an hour into the session, a strange phenomenon began to unfold. Lillian's body began to arch up, convulse and twist. She cursed the people around her in a deep man's voice. She struggled free from the acupressure of some of the people holding her.

They continued the session as instructed by Dr Ray. Then Dr Ray himself announced he would need to do another exorcism. With a loud and commanding voice, he decreed, 'In the name of Jesus, Saint Germain and all the ascended masters, I command the entity in this body to leave now and go directly to the light of God!'

Immediately, a strong wind blew upwards out of her body. The people directly around her had their hair blown straight upwards. Myself and the people around me had our hair blown backwards. The wind was felt across the room. It freaked the f**k out of everybody. People screamed and ran out of the building, shouting, 'Where is it going next!' while others climbed out windows or huddled in a corner.

Lillian's body then calmed down and she casually got up and walked into the bathroom. You could hear a pin drop. People began to cry and cuddle. There was no debate or attempt to explain what we had just seen and felt. Lillian emerged from the bathroom to declare that the scars on her temples from when she'd had shock therapy had disappeared. Apparently, there are thieves in the spiritual world that will try to steal a place in your body if your spirit is knocked or shocked out.

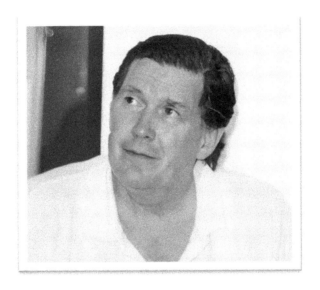

The amazing Dr John Whitman Ray discussing
Body Electronics

The Body Electronics meetings were usually held once a week at the hall of the local spiritual centre. Some of us who were very keen would also gather at the homes of practice facilitators another couple of days a week. I was attending one of these community sessions when I experienced some other strange phenomena.

A group of us heard drumming from one of the rooms and upon investigation, learned that an ex-drummer from Johnno's Blues Band was having acupressure and was somehow releasing suppressed sounds. It seemed to echo in the ether around his body, when in fact it was coming out of his body. Again, from another room, we smelled burning flesh, only to find the woman having acupressure was apparently re-living her children being burned in a war camp.

We came to understand that our cells carry memory and these memories can be passed on from one life or generation to another. A bit like when every cell in our body changes every seven years, yet because of cellular memory, a scar does not disappear. Rather than causing me fear or confusion as some would imagine, I believe that these types of experiences have afforded me greater fortitude, calmness and acceptance of the realities of our existence.

It was during the same session that I had my most personal experience with Body Electronics. We had been taught that there was an order to follow concerning particular acupressure points; otherwise, we would get ahead of where we should be in our healing. Dr Ray was not present, and the facilitators had become relaxed in their discipline that night. I was being held in a few different acupressure points, including one reserved for after full physical healing had occurred, which was not my case. It was my third eye point or pineal gland.

After about twenty minutes of sustained acupressure between my eyes, I had a profound experience that plunged me into a deep meditative-like state. Though I had my eyes closed, it was like somebody had turned a pink flood light on. I lost perception of my body weight and it was as though I was floating. I had a feeling of bliss from the tip of my toes to the top of my head. They had apparently activated the pineal gland.

Each time I tried to close my eyes, the sensation of bliss became magnified so much that I had to open my eyes again. The main facilitator and his daughter eventually had to take me to a disability facility and nurse me. Two weeks later, I realised that I was not ready for this constant consciousness of bliss as I had much more work to do on Earth, not the least being the full healing of my body, and purposely decided to will it away. In an instant, I regained full consciousness and with that, the sensation of my body weight.

Here's also something interesting about the acupressure techniques I learned through the teachings of Body Electronics:

Unholey Teeth

Whether it was some food stuff caught between my teeth, too much sugar or maybe medications, I found myself one day with the beginning of tooth decay. I had known of people that had gotten a hole in their tooth, only to end up in excruciating pain for sometimes months, with occasionally the end result being them needing a root canal, costing a lot of money.

I remembered my teachings about acupressure and decided I would apply it to the hole in my tooth. Knowing that the majority of living things could only go without oxygen for around three minutes, I decided that the bacteria causing the hole in my tooth was no different. I found the most painful part and pushed to the edge of my pain tolerance. After those three intense minutes, I let go. A rush of blood came flooding back to the area, seemingly flushing the poison from the rotting area. I felt I was onto something.

The simple fact that I was pressing hard at that place gave my body the understanding that I was not accepting what was happening there. I surmised that even if I damaged some gum, it was still better than losing the tooth for life. Besides, sometimes gums were affected by a rotting tooth and the process may deaden the nerve of the gum, which would stop any associated pain, with the gum eventually growing back.

I continued to apply acupressure to the most painful part of the hole in my tooth three times a day for three days. I woke up the day after to find the hole was gone.

There have probably been about eight occasions in my life when a hole started to form in my tooth, and I fixed it with this method. A couple of times the hole seemed inaccessible because it was inside my tooth. I overcame that problem by loosening off that tooth, grinding down on a bit of rubber. The resulting rush of blood to the area always flushed away any tooth decay-causing bacteria, with the tooth healing back in place. At fifty-four years of age, I have never needed a filling.

Bringing the SWAT Team to Their Knees

I became a volunteer in local organisations and found there needed to be a stronger voice for people with disabilities in the region. I decided to establish a group and eventually founded the first advocacy incorporation in Cairns for people with disabilities. The job had both moments of triumph and times of challenge. Believing in giving everybody a fair go, I allowed all people to nominate for positions on our committee, including people with physical and intellectual disabilities.

We routinely had three rounds of votes to pass what would normally be passed in one. The first one sometimes passed without a hitch but sometimes a committee member voted against something, like approving the allowed travel expenses to and from meetings. 'Harry is not allowed to get back his taxi fare because I don't like his hat!' was one particular incident. By the second vote, after heckling and prompting by carers, parents or advocates, the vote usually changed to positive. We still had the third one for good measure.

After declaring the close of the meeting one day, I unconsciously verbalised my thoughts of a trip to the pub. Straight away there were a lot of raised voices declaring they were going to the pub too. There were a few glares from parents as I realised what I had set off. As I rolled out, a hand reached out to catch a tow on the back of my chair. The next person latched onto the last person as a single file of wheelchairs, walkers, hoppers and every other kind of disability followed.

As we reached the intersection before the pub, the light turned red for us to wait. Sandy, who had down syndrome, yelled out, 'I'll pull the old disabled trick!' and promptly walked out into the middle of the traffic and stopped all the cars like a traffic cop. Cars screeched and all of them stopped. She waved us on, and we hung our heads in embarrassment as we scuttled across. The people in the pub could see us coming a mile away. As we turned through the glass doors into the lounge, chairs parted like the red sea to allow us through to the garden bar. We had no intention of going to the garden bar and headed straight for the main bar. Suddenly, there was a sea of red faces.

As a group, we applied for funding and it was granted. In the middle of 1992, with the grant, we opened an office and employed people to perform everyday duties. We helped to get ramps into buildings and up road curbs, arranged for appropriate pedestrian crossings and did an audit of all local hotels. I became acutely aware of the widespread lack of basic funding for the care of many people in difficult situations.

At one stage, I'd had enough. I had written, reasoned and represented to the point of frustration. It was now time to take action. I wrote to the local minister and threatened to chain her in her office while I protested out the front. I also told her that I headed an alliance of groups that would disrupt the up-coming Community Cabinet Meeting being held locally in Gordonvale.

At around 7 p.m. a few nights later, which was the night before the Community Cabinet Meeting, I was lying down on the bed in the lounge room of my mum's unit. I had been staying there temporarily while my live-in carer was on holi-day. The bed was a fold-out from the lounge and therefore very low to the ground. A loud knocking at the door startled both Mum and me. Opening the door, we were even more surprised to see the SWAT team. There were at least six of them in full bullet-resistant body suits, armed with machine guns. They yelled that they were there to 'Speak with Mr Innes' and demanded entry, to which we did not resist, of course.

They then began to demand that I not disrupt the Com-munity Cabinet Meeting. Having thought that they were there because of some danger in the vicinity, I was bewildered. I told them if they wanted to talk to me, I refused to have them look down on me and they would need to get on their knees beside my bed.

Disgruntled, but with no recourse, they reluctantly kneeled. I then told them that they should hand over the cheque that the minister had obviously written for the people needing care. They said they had no such thing and asked again that I do not disrupt the Community Cabinet Meeting. I told them that I was within my rights to protest, and they were pathetic errand boys. I said that if they did not leave immediately, I would contact the media and embarrass the politician who'd sent them. They themselves would be shamed and sacked for such a show of force against someone simply trying to help people with disabilities.

They asked who were the other groups that were aligned with me. I told them I would not tell them and to get out now. They left like sad little puppies, and I commented that they were very big men and hope they slept well that night. They never mentioned chaining the minister into her office; I think they didn't like her as well. There was never any alliance of groups, just me. My mum was used to my fighting spirit and knew nothing of the letter. After they left, she simply said, 'Would you like a cup of tea, love?'

After being involved in the establishment and on the committees of some other groups, I began travelling the country to attend seminars. I was asked to lecture in different institutions, including the hospital for student nurses on the subject of disability itself, and the local university on voluntary involvement in community organisations. I was offered a degree as a social worker if I did one year of study at the university. I felt I had no need to obtain a piece of paper to do what I was already doing.

I decided I would visit a man named William, just a couple of streets away from my own home. He had an injury similar to mine and had asked me to drop in sometime. While there, I met his live-in carer, Gerald. They both seemed pleasant, and I asked them to call on me if they ever needed assistance or advice. The next morning, I received a phone call from William telling me that Gerald had stolen his last ten dollars and disappeared at midnight. I was furious that a person would do such a thing.

A month or so later I happened to need to visit the X-ray department of the Cairns Hospital for my regular abdominal scans as a person with a spinal injury. I noticed Gerald out of the corner of my eye. He was limping towards reception. I told my mum to stay put while I snuck away to phone the police.

As I waited outside the department for the police hidden from the entrance, I saw Gerald leave. I told my mum he was not getting away and to tell the police I was following him. He left the hospital and headed north. I hung back and hid in my power wheelchair behind parked cars. I felt like an elephant trying to tippy-toe. He turned a corner, and I raced there so as not to lose him. I could see him but there was a big open space between us, so I waited. After a while, he turned another corner. By the time I got there, he was gone. I knew he had to live on that street. Just then, the police pulled up beside me. I told them they were too slow.

Another month later, I was at the hospital again getting my results. I couldn't believe my luck, but there Gerald was again. This time I would surely get him. I rang the police and used some strong demands. They arrived quickly and told me to wait outside. When the police emerged, they told me they could not arrest him right now as he was about to have an operation, though they assured me they would as soon as they could. I said to them that unless they waited there until after the operation, he would escape. On my subsequent enquiry, I learned that he had indeed escaped.

Several months went by when a friend relayed a story to me about money being stolen from his house. He showed me a picture of the culprit whom he had known as a friend. Who else was it but Gerald? I told him my story, and we marched to the police station. We were astounded to see that the only identikit photo on the wall was Gerald. We charged a young policeman with the job and told him we would hound him until this man was arrested. For two years we enquired about the case. We were delighted to receive a phone call one day to hear that Gerald had finally been arrested. He was not only wanted for theft but the rape of a person with a disability. He was sentenced and jailed for six years.

The Mary Poppins Stunt

The local shopping centre was only about ten minutes' drive in my electric wheelchair from my government-subsidised house in Earlville, a suburb of Cairns. I would often go there by myself for groceries. On this particular day, the sky had become overcast but I decided to chance it anyway and took off. After having done my shopping, with a few bags hanging off the back of my chair, the rain started coming down heavily. Taxi waits were sometimes half an hour or more, so I decided to buy a big-ass umbrella that would cover me, the groceries and the electrics.

I managed to lodge the umbrella between my leg and the side of the seat, then set off to cross the busy highway that was adjacent to the shopping centre. The light went green for me to cross. I was smack bang in the centre of the road when a sudden gust of wind hit me. The umbrella stuck fast and my whole chair lifted and tilted to its side, with only the two left wheels touching the ground. It looked cool, just like the stunt cars do it. For me, it was not cool. I continued forward for a few feet when the wind picked up and started to drag me sideways, still on two wheels but towards the traffic coming from the other direction. The umbrella was pulling upwards, so I didn't actually tip over. A few scary seconds passed before the traffic saw me and managed to stop. Luckily the wind slowed down too, and my wheelchair dropped back onto its four wheels. I hastily dislodged the umbrella and waved thank you to the traffic.

The sky darkened further as dusk approached. I was on the last stretch home, a road with a long straight, which then turned as it ascended a hill, and the crest had a railway crossing. Now, I knew that the best place for me to cross the railway was in the middle of the road, where it was the least bumpy, so I headed up the hill and looked around to make sure no cars were in sight. All was clear as I headed towards the middle of the road and carefully began to cross the railway. I was only halfway across when suddenly the wheelchair stopped. The lights were out, and I banged on as many parts as I could reach. She was dead.

Because of the way the road was, it would be difficult for a car to see me until it was too late, or I could get cleaned up by a train. The fading light added to the danger. My immediate thought was to launch myself onto the road and army crawl the hell out of there. As I contemplated my fate, I could see a few young kids walking on the footpath next to the road and coming my way. They seemed to be only five or six years old.

I muttered to the universe that if somehow these kids rescued me, then I would donate the wheelchair to the disabled children's home.

'Are you okay, mister?' they yelled out.

Just then, the lights on the chair turned back on. 'I am now but thank you!' I yelled back.

About a week after delivering the wheelchair to the disabled children's home, I thought I would ring the government and tell them I needed a new chair. When they found out what I had done with the last one, they said that they would pretend they did not hear what I had just told them, and that could I not give the next one away. I did. The sweet old lady needed it more than I did.

In Spirit & in Truth

About four years after my injury, my father passed away. He had battled cancer for years and finally lost his fight. He was well-loved, respected and missed by all. A couple of months later, in the middle of the night, I couldn't sleep and happened to open my eyes. The spirit of my dad was standing in my room, softly smiling at me. He appeared as his 19-year-old self. The only reason I recognised him was from a photo when he was young because he had his famous greasy-looking hair-do, the 'Bondi Wave', characterised by the generous helping of Brylcreem. My initial reaction was to ask him what he wanted. There seemed to be a slight time delay before he realised I could see him. He looked surprised and then faded away. I came to realise later on, through my own spiritual experiences, that our spirit understands that it should not interfere with anybody else's karma or evolution of spirit.

Up until that time, I fluctuated from being inspired and focusing on healing, clean living and extreme health routines to periods of defeat and self-pity, turning to things like drinking and smoking dope. After the experience of seeing my father's ghost, I focused on good health again as I began to consider the spirit and its eternal truth.

One night when I was lying in my bed, feeling uncomfortable and restricted, I found myself, as many able-bodied people also do, unable to sleep. But I could not just roll over, get up and make myself a cuppa, have a bath or go for a walk. I couldn't do anything but lie there. I was forced to contemplate my reality, and reality on many levels, asking the big questions. I thought on my personal problems, of those around me and the world at large. So great was my desire to free myself and my world of its problems that I gave myself the ultimate challenge: to have power over my spirit. To attempt to separate my spirit from my body.

I had many trials and failures, but I did eventually conquer my spirit and later taught people how to travel in their own spirit, meeting them face to face in the astral world. A place that is in the same time and has the same physical characteristics as this world, but in a spiritual dimension. A place where we are also creating our own universe through our desires, dreams and visions.

I have continued to teach people how to travel in their spirit throughout my lifetime, using this understanding to also help ghosts move on and clear spaces of negative energy. Through the seeming misfortune of becoming a quadriplegic,

I found the wisdom that has given me the treasure of experiencing our true nature, our eternal spirit and freedom. I've decided to include a small section on spirit travel towards the end of this book.

Squashing My Balls

It was 1992 and I was back in the comfort of my own home. A delightful young man by the name of Kyle had begun caring for me, and we encouraged each other in a healthy and spiritual lifestyle. I had begun sharing with him my technique for spirit travel and attempting to meet him each night on the astral plane. One morning he was very excited to tell me that he had indeed remembered our encounter in the spirit world the night before. I truly felt that this was the most powerful thing that I had done and could ever do with another human. It set me on a lifelong path of continued passion to meet people in the spirit world.

It was my carer Kyle's day off, and he had decided that he would go skydiving. As he walked casually across the lounge room, he announced his intentions and asked if anybody would like to go with him. Immediately, his girlfriend Laili said that she would like to go. I looked at my carer Keirryn and commented that I was jumping on the bandwagon. Keirryn said that I was crazy, and she would not do it. Excitement and adrenaline overrode any fear that I may have had and I decided to go anyway.

The parachuting company informed us that it was entirely possible for a quadriplegic to jump out of a perfectly good plane. The head instructor said that he had jumped with people with spinal injuries before. We paid top price to go as high as we could and received a short training session at the airport. The training included moving to the door of the plane, waiting for the count to three and then a simulated jump. As the plane seemed to be the smallest aircraft I had ever seen, only two jumpers and their tandem person could fit in at once. I decided I would watch Kyle and Laili first and then do my jump.

Keirryn and I drove to the field where Kyle and Laili were to land. We watched them float down happily and then touch down like ballerinas. Everything seemed like it went to plan, and I was keen to go. Back at the airport, my tandem instructor and I shuffled into the back of the plane and did a last-minute gear check. The plane took off and soon we were at 14,000 feet, and the field where we were to land looked as big as a matchbox.

We shuffled to the door, and I waited for the count. Suddenly, without counting, we were out the door. I didn't have time to take a breath. We were falling through the sky at lightning speed with my tandem instructor strapped to my back and the wind pressure from underneath pushing so hard on my chest that I was unable to breathe. It seemed like forever but eventually, the instructor pulled the rip cord and our parachute deployed. Though I had my knees bent up and strapped to my chest, the leg straps slid up and were squashing my balls. The instructor was yelling out, 'How did you like that?' Still gasping for air, all I could think was that he was an arsehole for not counting. I do admit that I did enjoy the last part of the jump when we were floating around like birds, despite my balls.

A couple of big guys had been organised to help catch us as we landed. We flew straight past them at speed and were heading towards an area of long grass. About ten metres above the ground, the wind changed, and we dropped straight down. We touched the ground with considerable force as the instructor flipped over the top of me. We continued to violently flip over each other a couple more times. We finally stopped with our legs and arms all over the place.

Kyle raced over and picked me up straight away. He asked me if I was okay, and I told him that I thought I may have broken a rib. He gingerly carried me to our car. I had severe pain every time I took a breath. I immediately went to see my osteopath, who reassured me that I had no broken bones. Three days later, I burped profusely and apparently dislodged the compressed air that had been in my lungs. The pain disappeared. After that, I tried to stop doing things which could so easily once again break my neck.

The Appreciation Celebration

The Tablelands area where I sustained my spinal injury was promoted by the local government and businesses as a popular swimming spot for locals and tourists alike, with detailed maps showing a way to get there. A feature of the map included crossing a railway line and some stairs to descend. The local council also promoted the area by beautifying the gardens in the immediate vicinity.

It is in fact illegal to cross railway lines without a designated crossing and the stairs, even though they were concrete, were apparently construction stairs built only for establishing the weir. At the top of the stairs was a sign that read 'NO SWIMMING ACCESS WITHIN 30 METRES OF THE WEIR GATE.' This, I said, suggested to me that it was safe to swim more than 30 metres from the weir gate.

The day before my injury, it had been raining, and the water was even murkier than its usual muddy brown. The various high-water marks on the rock from where I entered made it impossible to determine the latest level. On top of this, a local politician had decided it was a good idea to let the water out of the weir to cause a waterfall over the Barron Gorge, allowing tourists to see it from the Kuranda Train. This was initiated without consulting the public or letting any of the locals know.

So, what would have been an ordinary swim across the weir became a swim into a rock, which was now four feet higher underneath the surface of the water due to the drop in the water level. As a regular swimmer there, I knew the normal depths. Notwithstanding this, I still should have checked for logs or rocks that could have been washed down the river.

I could still, however, hold the government to its own laws. For six years, I prepared my case. Every day I did something towards it. I gathered references of my character, work records, statements from witnesses, photos taken by friends on the day of the accident and newspaper articles with photos from the air. It was at this time that I joined committees, started new community organisations and took a training job with the government. During all that time, I was flat broke.

At one stage, a First Nations friend of mine told me he was upset with me because due to my court case, the government had killed all the fish. He said they had drained the weir at midnight and blew up the rock that I had my injury on with TNT to destroy the evidence. On being informed of this allegation, my solicitors, barrister and QC gave up. They said we had no chance against such determination. They did not know me. I would not give up because of intimidation.

102

I decided I would start by taking out the opposition's main witness, the local policeman. He was the first government employee on the scene and therefore, their main witness. I'd heard some negative rumours about his character, so I sought to find evidence against him to discredit him. Fortunately, as a young man before my injury, I was involved in some voluntary community organisations that were now to serve me well. I recalled attending a community meeting in Kuranda, which was organised to protest against recent police brutality. At the same time, the police were holding a meeting at the RSL hall.

At our meeting, a panel of community representatives sat facing the crowd. It was announced that people that had been arrested for one reason or another had also routinely been assaulted before being locked up. Now it had happened to some well-respected First Nations Elders. The community was in uproar and the meeting was attended by all walks of life. A few people gave testimony of their own harrowing experiences. They all sounded the same to me and it seemed as though the meeting would go nowhere.

As a teenager and being relatively new to town, I felt it was not my place to speak. I subsequently said to my girlfriend Gypsie, 'I know what I would say,' and announced that I wanted to leave. She immediately raised her hand and announced, 'Happy has something to say.'

I was asked to come up the front. I had a very bright coloured shirt on and now my face was the same colour. I proposed that we formed 'what Barry said' the 'Kuranda Liberty Committee'. However, our constitution would be that

'We the undersigned reserve the right to be contacted at the time of arrest of any other member of the Kuranda Liberty Committee.'

I argued this could prevent the assaults between the time of arrest and the time of incarceration. Turning to the present police liaison officer, I asked if this was legal. He said he believed it was. With that, I announced I would now sit down and write that short constitution, and those who wanted to could come and sign underneath. Just then, my girlfriend's mother shouted out, 'Nice shirt, Paul!' and there was both laughing and clapping. I did not know if the crowd was laughing and clapping at her joke and me and my shirt, or at what I had just suggested. I sat down to write and to my delight, the crowd got up and lined up to sign. I quickly handed over the reins to a prominent First Nations Elder and the Kuranda Liberty Committee was born.

I never thought about it again until I was trying to work out how to discredit the policeman. But now I remembered that he was a main figure of the protest at the time. Because I now lived in Cairns, I decided to ring my old mate Dave who still lived in Kuranda, whom I had spent much time around while involved in the theatre and knew that he was well-informed in Kuranda community affairs. I asked Dave if the Kuranda Liberty Committee still existed.

'I am the president,' he said. The group's name had been changed to Kuranda Citizens Liaisons Committee and had apparently become a model for the state.

I asked him if he knew of anybody that had dirt on the particular policeman. Dave told me there was a young First Nations dancer that had had him investigated by the Criminal Justice Commission. I consequently approached the young man and asked him if he would sign a letter having the investigation information released to me. He agreed and a few weeks later a large parcel arrived on my doorstep. The policeman had been investigated by more than one tribunal and reprimanded. I highlighted those facts and hired a secretary. Her job was to come to my barrister's office and slam the papers down when I gave her the nod. My barrister was amazed that I had got such information. I demanded he get back on the case and ring the solicitor's firm in front of me, to which he did.

My employer Geoff had written me a great reference that mentioned my job, skills, community involvement and most importantly for me, the suicide of Gypsie. From day one, my legal team told me they did not want to use it. They said because he was overseas and could not be contacted, the judge might think the author was fictitious. They argued that while I was working, I was on the dole and that I had also not paid tax in two years. They said that the judge would see me as dishonest and would probably not even believe me that my injury had occurred in the way I described it or the place I said it did. I told them that was ridiculous and I would hand it up. We argued about the point every time we met until the day we entered court.

I am not permitted by law to disclose the events of the actual court case; suffice to say that the opposition was forced to begin out-of-court settlement negotiations before lunch that day. I was told to go home and wait for an offer and after a couple of days of tough negotiations, a settlement was made to the satisfaction of all parties.

Many people had helped me since my injury, so I decided to throw a free concert. On January 7th, 1994, I had the 'Appreciation Celebration', where 3,500 people turned up to the Kuranda Amphitheatre. There were a dozen local performers, a free bar, child minding, entertainment for the children and long tables of rare organic exotic tropical fruit.

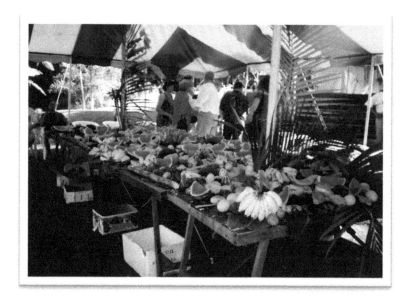

A table of organic fruit at the Appreciation Celebration.

I must have looked tired at the end of the day because appearing from nowhere was around half a dozen little fairies.

They seemed to be in their early teens and were probably the daughters of some of my friends. They informed me that they were taking me for a rest. With that, they picked me up and carried me to my marquee, where they had covered my mattress in flowers. They lay me down and all began to massage me. I was asleep in seconds.

The Natural Love Sanctuary

Still living in a government-provided house in suburbia, I now began the pursuit of my own property. My family, friends, carers and I talked about our options. We had exhausted the block where we were living with thirty-five fruit trees and various abundant veggie patches and herb gardens. Continuing my focus on health and healing, I surrounded myself with a group of fellow raw foodists. Every day, a bunch of us met at lunchtime in the backyard for a big raw salad, exotic and delicious seasonal fruit and to think about our best course of action.

I had met a man named Lance at Body Electronics and again at some spiritual groups. He seemed like a nice guy and told me about the property he owned. His dream was for it to be a self-sufficient community, a sanctuary for healing, free for all to come. I thought that was groovy and I'd had the same sort of dream for a property of my own for a long time. Sometime just before my settlement, Lance had asked me to come and visit one day, so I did. I arrived at the property about an hour and a half drive northeast of Cairns. It was semi-remote, being at the end of a dirt road and over some rickety bridges, through a forest and into an opening. It seemed like a beautiful oasis. There was an aura of peace about the place, yet it looked like a fairly run-down farm. I thought to myself, *If I ever had the money, I would never buy a place like this* as there was just too much work to do.

Lance rang me soon after the settlement and told me that the property was in eight shares, yet he could not find investors with the qualities he wanted and was about to lose the property to the bank. Having never had lots of money in my life, I was trying to help anyone and everyone with everything. I asked him to give me a little time and I would seek a cosmic sign to see if I was to come to the financial aid. A book lay in front of me during the phone call. It was called *Man of Miracles*. I silently prayed, 'Lord, if I go, will you come?' I opened the book to a random page. The first thing my eyes lighted down on was 'there was a forest and the Lord came.'

I had only ever intended to support Lance's dream financially, so I gave Lance a share to be the caretaker. His friends, Ben and Deirdre, had helped him with the property from the time he first acquired it, so I gave them a share and told them they could pay me for it whenever they could. The deed to them was worded 'out of love and natural affection'. It therefore, did not attract any stamp duty.

I had only been at the sanctuary for a few months when a young lady named Lucy, whom I had known when I was a teenager, came to visit the property. I soon got lost in her beautiful blue eyes, and we fell deeply in love. After spending some time together, I gathered my brother and three of my mates for a pre-planned trip to the Townsville casino. We decided we would fly down for the weekend, and I would pay all expenses with the $5000 I took, which was more money than I'd ever had or seen. We arrived, dropped off our luggage, and went straight to the gambling arena.

One of my friends and I saw some shirts for sale at a counter. They had the casino emblem on the pocket, and though they were daggy denim, we still decided to buy them for the novelty. We quickly went to our rooms and changed into them. Back in the casino itself, we decided to play the 'chocolate wheel' even though it was the worst odds for returns. My friend put the $10 maximum amount on my favourite number 47 for me, and then put $10 on the same number for himself, right next to mine. It came up, and we jumped for joy. Okay, I didn't jump.

The croupier announced that we had put double the maximum amount on and only one dividend would be paid. We protested, announcing that I could not reach the number from my wheelchair and that my friend had to do it for me. The croupier spoke to management and came back with the news that our declaration could not be verified and only one payment would be made. Without hesitation, I demanded that if we could not bet what we wanted in the main arena, we be allowed to enter the high rollers room. In truth, I did not know if such a place existed or if it was only to be found in Las Vegas or Hollywood movies!

The croupier once again consulted management. We were denied, and they cited our inappropriate attire. This time we had them. We told them we had bought the shirts from the casino. The croupier went red and yet again consulted management. They reluctantly agreed and we were escorted to a separate room and afforded the best service after they saw our wad of cash. I took the opportunity to smugly ask, 'Can I now please have my carers assist me?' They obliged because we seemed dumb and rich, and they did not want to discriminate against me. Little did they realise I had hatched a plan to tilt the odds in my favour with my new extra manpower.

Having an ex-girlfriend's cousin in the business of being a croupier, I understood that they could be trained to make the ball land on any number. Though the wheel was spinning, and the ball spun the other way, they knew where to place it and how hard to spin it, practising for months to get it right. I also knew that after they let go of the ball, they announced to punters 'last bets' before they would count to three under their breath and declare, 'no more bets'.

I knew that because there were 36 numbers and the zero, and the return was 35 to 1, we could potentially cover 35 numbers, leave out two numbers and still get a return of one extra chip. In the main gambling area, people put their chips on top of the other people's chips, so it was hard to move them in those last three seconds. But now, in the high rollers room, we had our own table. I took my team for a walk and told them I would give them a percentage of the winnings if they helped me with my plan. I told them to cover 80 or 90% of the board. After the ball was released and within those three seconds, they were to move the chips to cover the other numbers and therefore, the croupier would never know which number to drop the ball on. We won $47,000.

Because the management did not want us to leave, they offered us free accommodation, drinks and food for the rest of our stay. We were told that the only thing we would have to pay for was our phone calls and any movies we watched. We entered the casino the next day feeling like kings. Our run of luck continued and in the early hours of the morning, we fell exhausted onto our beds. As we were in a semi-sleep, adrenaline-pumped state of consciousness, we could see roulette wheels spinning and chips piling high.

At the first movement of anyone, we were all up and raring to go again. After a few nights of constant winning, we had now secured the presidential suite, an executive suite and three other rooms. I continued to divide the loot with my team as our partners, family and other friends arrived. Even though we were winning big, I could still not get shoes on my down-to-earth girlfriend, Lucy. After a week, it was finally time to go home.

We booked the plane, our cabs and met in the lobby with packed bags. We were paying the bill for our phone calls and movies when I found a stray chip in my pocket. I took a carer into the gaming area only to find the cashier was on the opposite side of the room, so I placed the chip on the nearest table on an outside chance. It won. I moved the chips and won again. I did it again and won. Within a couple of minutes, I had turned it into $8,000. I gingerly told our crowd who were, of course, stunned. I announced I would hand an extra thousand dollars each to our team if everybody wanted to stay another week. After some discussion, we stayed.

We continued our streak of luck. Though we had free access to massage, saunas, restaurants and tennis courts, we were becoming pasty from staying indoors going from our room to the roulette table and back. We once again booked and packed to go. It felt like Groundhog Day when I found another chip in my pocket. Surely, I could lose this one on a ridiculous bet. Not so. I won $6,000. My crowd looked at me, some with sheer amazement and some with frustration. My team could not stay any longer as now they would not only lose their jobs, but also their partners. We had to go. The casino management offered to come and pick us up any time by Learjet and limousine. I have always thought about going back but never have because there always seemed to be something even more exciting or better to do with my life.

Coming back to the sanctuary, I stayed for a while and swam in the river every day, enjoying all the strange new fruits that I had never seen or even heard of. Before long, as most people do in life, I felt the urge to travel and explore my world.

A team of six of us, including Kyle and Laili, geared up and set off on an adventure around Northern Australia in my new four-wheel drive. This vehicle was no ordinary four-wheel drive. It was a 21-seat Mercedes Unimog truck with eight forward and reverse gears. I had it modified to include a double bed so Lucy and I could lay back and still see the road ahead. We stocked up, made some rough plans and headed off into adventure.

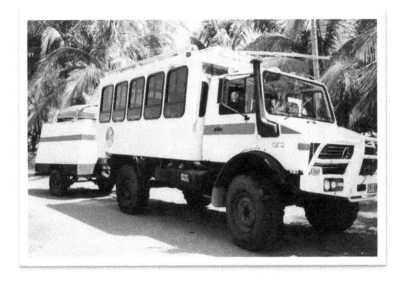

The Unimog with a bamboo pole on top for collecting coconuts, towing our trailer with a motorbike and handmade boat.

We reached Uluru in the Red Centre late one afternoon. It was hot and dry, and this great rock was imposing, a lone monolith with striking colours against a wide-open sky as the pink and golden sun went down. We decided we had missed too much before it got dark and would come back in a few days after visiting Alice Springs. During the time we were away, it had rained – a rare event in the area. On our return, a vast array of stunning wildflowers of every colour had sprung up throughout the whole desert surrounding Uluru. It was dreamlike and contrasting against a backdrop of the far distant horizons.

We explored many swimming holes on our travels and found ourselves stopping off in little outback towns so that we could help Lucy's little sister Emma with study and to sit her home-schooling tests, supervised by an approved local official.

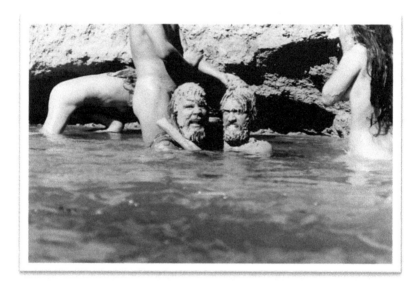

Hippibottomus in a swimming hole in the Northern Territory on our way around Australia.

Once we had reached Darwin, Lucy wanted for her and I to be able to enjoy some time together, away from other people. She said we had never been so close to another country as we were in Darwin and suggested we travel overseas to India. I was happy to be travelling with just my girl and was excited at the thought of the mysteries of exploring a foreign land. There was a particular guru that we had both become inspired by that we could also visit in India, whose name was Sai Baba. I wondered if Lucy would be able to take care of me being in a wheelchair, and somehow also shuffle our suitcase and a shower chair. She assured me that she would be more than capable.

An Ashram in India

I had never been overseas before and had no idea of how much it would cost. I bought $10,000 worth of Indian Rupee and $10,000 worth of traveller's cheques. We packed up the shower chair with our luggage and rolled off into the sunset.

On arrival in India, we were enchanted to see that it had a great spiritual richness, with yogis and babas everywhere in bright robes, smiling and laughing and offering profound wisdom to the passers-by. Its streets were alive with people, selling and performing, while the air was filled with ancient-smelling spices that I felt I recognised from a previous life.

But there was another side that we also began to see. We were shocked and saddened to see the vast poorness of some areas, with children maimed, having had their legs twisted around each other several times over a long period of time. Their disability could then earn money for their families or captors as these innocent children were forced to become professional beggars.

We decided to get out of the city and headed down south, inland, to stay at the ashram of Sai Baba in the little village of Puttaparthi. Experiencing what seemed to be a manifestation from the hand of Sai Baba, we were enchanted and felt we had witnessed real miracles. His discourses were infused with mesmerising mystical insights, and the daily duties and rituals were a sweet reprieve from the chaos of the outside world.

Each day we would venture out into a small town surrounding the ashram and be greeted by a group of children trying to sell us flower necklaces. I always bought one, apart from one day when I was in a hurry and had no money on me. That day, one of the little girls insisted I take a necklace as I hurried past. She said, 'You no pay.' I thought, *How sweet*, as I allowed her to place it around my neck. I thanked her and she immediately said, 'You pay tomorrow!' Scammed again.

We enjoyed our stay but after a couple of weeks, it was time for us to leave the ashram so we headed for the airport. We were waiting for our flight when I noticed three Indian people pointing at Australia on a world map. I approached them and asked if any were thinking of visiting Australia. One turned and said, 'Mate! I am Australian!' He had an Aussie accent and gave me a huge bear hug. The other two people were his brother and sister. His sister was from Germany and his brother was from Madras in India, where we were to fly to next for three days on our way home. They offered to be our hosts while we were there in Madras, and we humbly accepted.

After we arrived at the Madras airport, we followed them in our taxi to our accommodation. Motorists do not use blinkers in India. You get to merge into the other lane if you are beeping your horn the most, driving the fastest and looking the most aggressive or dangerous.

The next day, the two brothers offered to take Lucy and me on a taxi tour of their favourite holy sites. We started at the Church of Mary, which was on a beautiful beach. The church was empty, and they parked me right up next to the altar then walked away, disappearing into the back of the church. After some time, they seemed disappointed to see that I was not healed. We then drove to many different places, visiting the shrines of multiple Hindu gods. Each shrine had its own rituals, including chants and mantras, circling the large altar, putting ash on one's forehead or in one's mouth, offering gifts and lighting incense or candles.

The light was beginning to fade when we set off on yet another pilgrimage down many small lanes. I expressed that I was getting tired, and Lucy and one brother voiced a similar sentiment. The other brother insisted we see one last shrine as it was his favourite. He said we could stay in the taxi and he would do one circumference of the altar and return. We watched as he made his way around. He had nearly completed the circle when we saw a devotee of the resident guru approaching him as he shuffled along in his slippers. Our friend did not speak as the devotee whispered in his ear. His eyes lit up and he ran up to our taxi. He said, 'The guru, who does not usually see people in the night-time and with whom it ordinarily takes days to get an interview with, says, 'Bring the man in the wheelchair inside.'

The brothers looked at me strangely. Was I good or was I bad? I was wondering how he knew I was in a wheelchair. We had known our friend had not spoken to anybody and the wheelchair was still in the boot of the taxi.

I felt both intrigued and compelled to go inside. We rolled into what was a typical guru sight. A bearded and robed man sat in the lotus position, smiling. Soft music played, candles flickered and incense added a mirage-like sight. Lucy and I waited at the back of the room while he spoke to the brothers in Hindi. After a couple of minutes, they turned and one said, 'The guru says your injury is your desire to transmute the karma of your great-grandparents.'

That's typical, I thought, *sacrificing a lifetime to do somebody else's job for them.* Very nice of me of course, but ignorant after having come to understand that people must learn for themselves, and also pretentious in assuming they needed help. While I do actually believe in personal and collective karma, I also know that we can't help somebody else to evolve. We have an eternal pursuit of the harmonious balance of our existence, and it needs to come from the desire of our own spirit. No matter how much time passes, aeons and light-years, everything in the universe will correct itself. It is our individual conscience that judges us – our own morals and inner voice.

I was not born before all of my great-grandparents had passed. Maybe I was one of them, and had reincarnated, therefore trying to sort out my own stuff. How about I just consciously cancel it and forgive myself? Hey, presto! Nope, that didn't work. What the hell did they do anyway? Still, it gave me a reason to think on such. Also, from now on, I would make sure my karma did not run over my dogma.

We had a fascinating time in India, and upon leaving bought all manner of beautiful gemstones, jewellery and silks. On our return, we learned that the currency had changed 20% in our favour. When we cashed in the remaining Rupees and traveller's cheques, we had paid for our entire trip, everything we bought, and it also netted us a profit of $1500 on top. We were on a mission from God and did expect him to pick up the bill, but we didn't expect the tip!

The Sanctuary Becomes Self-Sufficient

Back at the sanctuary in Australia late in 1994, I was having a campout with my friends for my birthday and wanted to give myself a treat. I decided to hire a helicopter to fly my girlfriend Lucy, her little sister Emma and me from our sanctuary to Lucy's mother's place about 200 km away. The pilot took us on a route that passed behind Mt Bartle Frere, the third highest mountain in Queensland. He told us that we were flying over an area where there were so many waterfalls, the majority of them had never been named.

We flew to the bottom of some of the steeper falls, where we hovered and turned the helicopter vertical, then flew straight upwards! It was a great adrenaline rush. We then hovered at the bottom of mountains, angled the helicopter and flew straight up them just above the canopy until we reached the ridge when the land would suddenly drop away, and with it, our stomachs. I loved it but the girls were screaming too much, and the pilot and I decided we couldn't stand the noise anymore.

We could see a place to touch down, just near the house. We all agreed it was a good place to land but as we touched the ground, dirt blew up from everywhere and covered the house. Dozens of pot plants blew over. It was a great first impression.

The next time I was back at the sanctuary, I was approached by my friends Ben and Deirdre. They explained that they were experiencing some personal issues and had reluctantly decided to give me back their share. They again signed it over 'out of love and affection' and it again attracted no stamp duty. Soon after, Lance came to me and told me that his ex-wife wanted half of his share or she was moving there with her new partner, whom Lance did not like. He also said that a psychic had told him that he should be working with children on an island. Subsequently, he was off to join UNICEF and wanted to sell his share. To avoid the share falling into the wrong hands, I bought it back. I was now the owner of the whole property and a quadriplegic farmer.

The land was four kilometres from the highway, with two kilometres of bitumen and then two kilometres of dirt. We were at the end of the road, with no neighbours for miles, and at the beginning of the mountains, encompassed by the mighty and pristine Mary River to the left of us, and the crystal clear and sweet waters of Windmill Creek to the right. They met

about one kilometre from the front gate. World heritage rainforest and mountains encompassed the rear, while above us,
the Mary had natural bubbling spas and gently massaging waterfalls. There were ancient caves and paintings dotted along
its edges as it rose stately into wild and misty mountains.

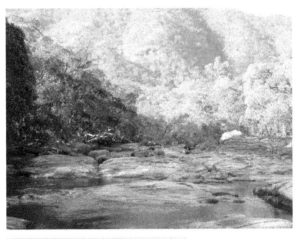

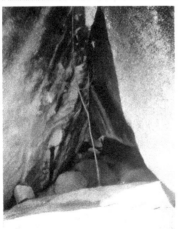

The Mary
A pristine source of
water and fish with
waterfalls and
natural spas. The
highest mineral
content was gold.

The Runaway Cave
Authentic First
Nations paintings
tell the story of two
forbidden lovers
that ran away from
their tribes to live
together in the cave.

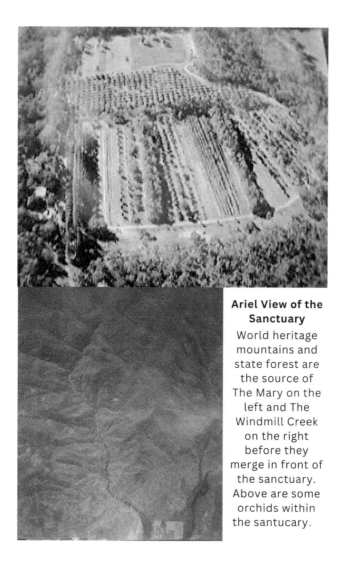

Ariel View of the Sanctuary
World heritage mountains and state forest are the source of The Mary on the left and The Windmill Creek on the right before they merge in front of the sanctuary. Above are some orchids within the santucary.

The property was eighty-eight acres, with thousands of organic fruit trees, paddocks, various houses, huts and sheds, including a very spacious community hall and a large library of fascinating books that had been donated. Some of the trees were eighty years old and bore hundreds of fruits, with their roots reaching down to the water table.

There were many that fruited all year round like the golden dwarf coconuts, the many types of citrus, papaws or the thousands of bananas. Various types of mango ensured that the hundreds of trees fruited for many months. There were four mulberry seasons per year and many dozens of rare exotic tropical trees such as rollinia, which tasted like custard; aki nut, which tasted like cheese and melted on a hot potato; and ice cream bean and chocolate pudding fruit, which were aptly named.

We had avocadoes, macadamia nuts, cotton bushes and one of the largest and oldest neem tree plantations in the southern hemisphere. Neem transmutes the positive ions in the air, the pollutants, more than any other tree known to mankind. It is also an anti-bacterial, anti-inflammatory, anti-fungal, anti-septic and anti-viral. It can be used as a natural pesticide and for many products, including toothpaste. Just planting the tree itself keeps away sand flies and mosquitos. In the heart of the land, a pink lotus pond glistened.

Aside from all these positives, there was much to be done to realise the sanctuary's full potential. There was a valley that was used as a rubbish dump by the previous owners, machinery was scattered throughout the property, tools were housed in various locations, building material lay on the ground here, there and everywhere, buildings needed renovation, fences needed fixing and everything needed pruning, mulching and better irrigation.

I began to gather the troops. Friends and visitors could see the possibilities and decided to help. I hired some workers and joined a farm stay network called W.W.O.O.F. (Willing Workers On Organic Farms.) They were people from all around the world willing to do four hours of work a day in exchange for their food, accommodation and to have a different cultural experience.

Modifying my trusty ride-on lawn mower, I was ready to start work. We picked up all of the rubbish in a gigantic valley on the land that was used as the rubbish dump, housed the machinery and tools in one place, made racks for the building material, renovated the buildings that needed it, fixed the fences and pruned every tree. We traced the kilometres of irrigation, digging some in and digging some out. We built a new causeway at the entrance to the property and strengthened the gates. Then we graded roads and began to plant veggie patches and herb gardens.

Replacing the mulch and keeping it regularly turned helped to break it down with just the right amount of microbes needed to do the job. Leaving mulch unturned regularly would cause larger bugs to come to eat the microbes, with cockroaches coming to eat them, spiders coming to eat them, rats coming for them, snakes coming for the rats and pigs coming for the snakes. It's all a food chain. Through this simple mulch maintenance and keeping building material off the ground, we gave no place for vermin to thrive and therefore we were able to create a true sanctuary where children could play safely and parents could relax.

We were at the perfect elevation from sea level, so it was never too hot or cold. I never used to sweat and could wear no shirt till midnight most of the year-round. We were the closest property to the mountains, so the air was fresh and the all-season river water that ran by us was pristine and sweet. The soil was well-drained and we were able to create new, rich soils in lots of areas from the breaking down of mulch. Everything we planted thrived.

The communal area included the community hall, a tool shed, a fruit packing shed, a schoolroom and surrounding gardens. Basic bulk food supplies, along with essentials like toilet paper and first aid, were kept there for guests and general community use. Permanent residents still had their own private houses, shacks or camps and everybody respected each other's personal spaces.

The property was now our home, and we were a self-sufficient community of up to sometimes forty people. We gave it the name of Mary River Mountains Sustainable Living Sanctuary. It was a bit of a mouthful so it eventually became The Natural Love Sanctuary.

Everything around us seemed to be associated with Mary. Our town was named Maryfarms, our river was the Mary and we lived on East Mary River Road. Even our scarecrow was named Scary Mary. Jamming was a regular occurrence at the sanctuary and before long we had a main group that played well together. Being health freaks, we loved to make jokes about society's meat heads, yobbos and junk food eaters. An ongoing laugh was about the number of hormones in processed food and how chicken, especially, was known to make males grow breasts and women moustaches. This joke, the surrounding Marys and the fact that we all sported some sort of beard at the time gave arise to the band's name, Hairy Mary.

My mum once told me why she had changed her middle name from Mary to Maria. She said that Mary was too 'woggy'. I told her that Maria was way more 'woggy' than Mary.

She said, 'Not where I was from; every second wog was named Mary!'

I was visiting my mum one day when I happened to mention the band. Mum looked at me, shocked. 'You know what we used to call our Hairy Mary?'

I was stunned. I had bad visualisations.

I mentioned the historical meaning of 'Hairy Mary' to the band. The next note we played was sour. The band began to fall apart. After that I called Mum, 'HM.' I told her it stood for Her Majesty.

Many people came to our sanctuary over time, seeking healing or rejuvenation. There were those that needed simple social acceptance, which was normal and freely given in our small community. Over time, they found themselves drawn naturally into the community and were able to empower themselves individually again. There were also those that had emotional, psychological or physical need of healing. We gave them love, space and good food.

The only money that we needed to survive was a small amount for rates, maintenance of the property, savings for upgrades, and to spoil ourselves every now and then. Money was never an issue, and we truly felt we were living a rich and carefree lifestyle. When you genuinely experience that all your basic needs are being met freely, everything else is a blessing of luxury. The way the modern world has people living in a housing estate is unnatural, and the average person has forgotten what self-sufficiency does for personal empowerment. In a self-sufficient community, there is no dog-eat-dog desire for power or fame. There is also no need to study a career that we are not personally interested in or does not benefit our life directly.

Therefore, for instance, we found ourselves some days happily deciding to spend the whole day swimming up the river. A large tribe of us would set off, some naked, carrying food for everybody, instruments and a stretcher to take me through some of the narrow paths on the way to the natural spas and waterfalls. Other days, a group would sometimes grate our coconuts to make coconut cream, rob our bees for honey, collect the macadamia nuts, chocolate pudding fruit and ice cream bean fruit, combine it all together to make a chocolate mousse-type sweet. All manner of people would line up in a long single file for their share.

Rusty's markets in Cairns was a favourite place for me to visit, where some of the exotic tropical fruit was so rare that I could only get it if I was one of the first people to turn up before dawn in some cases. The myriad of buskers scattered around made for an enchanting experience. One day a group of young teenagers approached me. One of them asked, 'Hey mister, you know your cult?'

'What?' I said as I was taken aback.

'You know, all the people wearing white.'

I looked around to realise that indeed not only I was wearing white, but a number of people in my party. At the time, I had become obsessed with everything being as natural as possible and because I knew that our skin absorbs, I was always wearing natural material that had not been dyed or bleached. To me, it was just my lifestyle, but to onlookers I understand now that we must have looked like a cult! I amusingly informed the young man that we were not a cult, but I did know the people that he was talking about.

'Well, we've heard that you don't take drugs and we was wonderin' if you would help us?'

Of course, I wanted to help these kids. Without too much thought of possible things that could go wrong, I decided I would take them in my big truck up to the sanctuary.

The experience seemed like it was therapeutic to them and though I couldn't get them to do anything too productive, I did feel it was helping them by keeping them away from the city and drugs. They stayed for a while and continued to come back and forth. Whenever they were there, it wasn't long before they wanted to head back to the city to collect their unemployment benefits and binge on junk food.

After an incident involving a candle being left to burn unattended in the community hall in the night-time, the resulting burn mark on the wooden bench got me thinking. We didn't have insurance, and I decided it was too risky to continue to allow the kids to come back and forth to the sanctuary. Once we had ferried the last one back to the city, I later learned of a similar situation on another property, whereby the whole property was accidentally burned down. I felt that I had averted potential disaster and realised that though I had the best intentions, it just wasn't possible to help everybody in every situation.

Around this time, I met a couple of men who were to become lifelong friends. Sahajo first came to the sanctuary in 1995 when he heard about our lifestyle while visiting his family in the area. He had grown up at nearby Mount Mulligan and was taught to be a tracker by the First Nations members of his family. He became an expert marksman, local boxing champion and prize-winning runner amongst many other things he did with his life, including serving in Vietnam and becoming a promoter, bringing the likes of Johnny Farnham, Kamal, Dinah Lee and many others to Cairns.

After seeking spirituality in his life, he mastered becoming a Buddhist monk and then eventually the security guard for some famous gurus around the world. On returning to Byron Bay, he took a different course and did stand-up comedy for a number of years. I like to tell everybody that I taught him everything he knows about his latest qualification as a tantric sex master. I recall one time that he was visiting Cairns and a tantric sex workshop was organised for him to teach. At the same time, he had managed to somehow be living at a nun's convent while teaching them yoga. I can only imagine what happened in the night-time. Sahajo's nature is sweet and kind, and he has always shared with me his wonderful wisdom and compassionate love. He has also just released his autobiography, *Gurus' Bodyguard*.

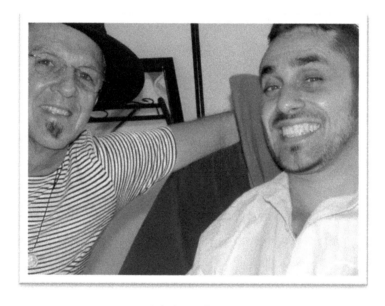

Sahajo and me.

At the same time, I was spending a lot of money at a local nursery in Mossman. Though I had never actually been myself, I had sent many people there to pick up things for me. The owner, Jed, was told about our sanctuary and decided he would come to visit me. Jed had taught horticulture at a local college and with my knowledge of organic farming, landscaping and experience with things like companion planting and permaculture, we found a lot in common and became good friends. Jed eventually came to live with me and even became one of my carers.

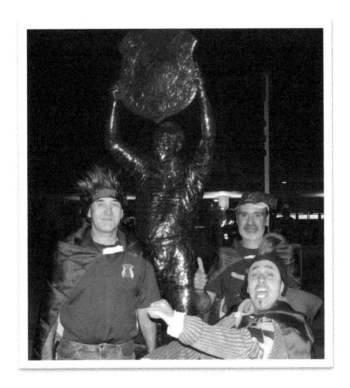

My brother Dan, my mate Jed and me when we won tickets to the State of Origin.

His selfless dedication to me over many years has touched me deeply. I've lost count of the times that he has physically saved my life. Times when my injury presented a complication and could have resulted in my death, Jed calmly took control. His genuine soul and gentle, patient temperament has been a guiding and stable light in my life. Jed also became close friends with my mum, and through the decades, we endured many struggles together. Though both of these men have led very different lives and have somewhat different natures, they have always been there for me, and I count them as my best friends.

The LSD Hitman

I had been at the sanctuary for just under a year. It was a few days after the new year had begun and we had some weary travellers arrive. They were a young couple that seemed meek and peaceful, and we welcomed them warmly. They set up a camp for themselves not far from the main community hall.

Everything seemed fine until a couple of days later when the young lady opened up to the other women about how her partner had taken LSD on New Year's Eve and had since then not seemed to regain his mental or physical composure. It had begun to take its toll on her when he continued to not get out of bed to even go to the toilet. She broke down and asked us what she should do. We rallied around her and began to take shifts caring for him. I myself decided to take him aside to try chanting to clear his mind and talk with him about general social psychology. It seemed to keep him peaceful at the time but there was no forthcoming depth of conversation.

A couple of days went by, and I was sunbathing by myself on the grass next to the community hall. I looked up to see him climbing a ladder that he had placed on the side of the building. We had a policy of no guns on the property, but I noticed that he had a rifle. Alarmed, I yelled for some help.

Somebody heard me, and I told them what was happening. By the time they got to the ladder, he was casually lying down on the roof and was pointing the rifle straight at me. Luckily the person was able to take the rifle from him and he did not resist. We questioned him on his motive for pointing the gun at me. He relayed that God had told him that two people had to die, and he had understood it was me first, then himself.

I knew a well-respected homeopath in Herberton. We decided it was our next move. It didn't seem to help him, and we felt we were out of ideas. His partner decided to take him back home to Melbourne. I was disappointed that we could not help him but happy to escape with my life once again.

Life went on as usual at the sanctuary. I had been with Lucy for a year and a half and had shared many wonderful experiences with her. One simple argument led to us parting ways. Later on in life, after visiting a clairvoyant, I realised I had not let go of Gypsie and had been sabotaging all of my relationships at the year and a half mark, the same amount of time that I had been with Gypsie.

As the months and years passed, I became acutely aware of the effect my mood would have on the forces of nature. It was no coincidence anymore. If I began to get angry about something, the wind would pick up or a nearby door would slam. If then I took no notice and stayed angry or got angrier over time, grey clouds would form, thunder would start to roll or animals would make wild calls. If still there was no resolve, the people in the sanctuary would start to argue, bushfires would threaten and strange and mysterious things began to happen. Calming my temper was the only refuge that the community had. When I had power over my emotions, there was sunshine, prosperity and the children laughed. I came to understand that we don't own land, the land owns us.

We became known to the region and the local women's shelter sent us women and children that needed refuge.

Many people abandoned their material possessions at our property and declared that they were out to become enlightened in the caves. Most were back within about four days. But some seemed to do just that, staying in the mountains for months, having no food, but coming and standing at our back gate from time to time, just to smile, with piercing clear eyes, naked and rosy-cheeked. None of them ever looked emancipated. Without speaking, one look from these radiant beings portrayed a thousand words and the immense power and true freedom of the human mind and body.

Australia's First Rainbow Gathering

Early in 1997 some people that I considered to be Elders rang me from Byron Bay. They were regular visitors to my sanctuary and told me that scouts for a 'Rainbow Gathering' were coming my way. The scouts were to ask me if I would allow a Rainbow Gathering to be held at the sanctuary. I was told by the Elders that the Hopi Indians had prophesied that one day a 13th tribe would wander the earth teaching the principles of sustainable communities, self-sufficiency and natural healing.

The gathering would be free and include workshops on a multitude of subjects. It would take place over the course of seven weeks: two setting up, three for the gathering itself, and two packing up. The Elders suggested that they would hold a circle to offer me their advice. I looked for my own sign, asking the heavens to send a chime if it were meant to be. In a nanosecond, somebody over in the next building dropped a large cooking pot, which chimed at about 100 decibels. The Elders also soon rang back and said it was a goer. The scouts told me that it had been a success in many places around the world, but this would be the first in Australia.

A magic hat would be passed around in the morning for donations, and it was always more than enough to pay for food and supplies. They said that they would do all the setting up, general management, cleaning and packing up afterwards. I tried to imagine myself sitting back and letting that happen. I said yes to The Rainbow Gathering and set out the conditions as some of the following:

Signs should be acknowledged before entry and all normal sanctuary guidelines would apply.

There will be no cars, dogs, electronic music or alcohol on the property.

There will be one entry and one exit point.

Sahajo used his charm and influence to get a permit for the gathering from the local council. Expecting a crowd of thousands, in July of that year around forty scouts, my team and I began some of the mammoth tasks needed to prepare. We built new composting toilets, kitchens and shower areas, along with growing live beds of food including about half an acre of sprouts. All advertising was word-of-mouth only. Luckily, I had continued to be involved in all areas of the organising because as the day approached, I realised that water had not been supplied properly to the amenities, and that I had to spend thousands of dollars immediately; otherwise, it would create unsanitary and unhygienic conditions.

The day finally arrived for the opening of The Rainbow Gathering. I was given a beautifully carved 'Talking Stick' to open the gathering. Many people began to arrive, and it seemed that there was now every kind of person under the sun at my doorstep. I eyed one girl in particular. I judged her and sighed at what I thought was a very peculiar clothing choice. The universe had humbled me by the end of the gathering after she decided to become my devotee, dedicating herself to my service and sleeping each night at my feet. A not-so-subtle lesson, pointing out how limiting and fickle our minds are if we believe we can evaluate a person in any way by their outward layer, whether it be skin colour, circumstance or clothes.

The main circle each day was focused around a huge fire pit. The first circle grew bigger until a thousand people were holding hands. There were gurus from India, federal government ministers with no shirts on, Hollywood movie stars, naked people, the local First Nations peoples, my family, friends, neighbours, carers, the W.W.O.O.Fers that were working at our sanctuary, the people who lived on our sanctuary, and it seemed people from every walk of life.

The concept was that the central fire pit would be the area where the main gathering would hold circles and initiate workshops, from meditation and healing circles to breakfast and donation circles, then talking and various workshops on disciplines, arts, crafts and lifestyle continuing until the dinner circle. Everything from preparing meals to washing dishes was done voluntarily. The Departments of Health and Environment taught workshops on waterway management and hygiene etc., and I especially enjoyed the workshops about the Mayan Calendar and the one on the many uses of Aloe Vera. 24-hour cafes offering free chai scattered our property, and the soft beat of drums put the whole valley into a peaceful sleep every night.

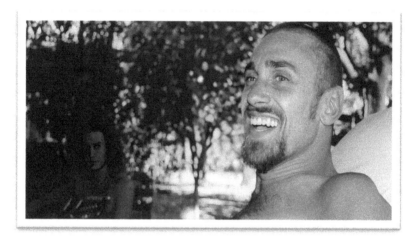

My heyday jamming with my mate, Jef.

After a few days camped near the main circle, I was the only one still camped in the middle of the paddock, enduring the dry heat of the day and the still cold of the night. Every other person had to retreat beyond the tree line. Though I had my main house, another house on the river, a full-sized liveable mobile wagon and even lived in the community hall from time to time, I decided it was time to go back to my main camping spot in the sanctuary, near the river in the north-east. I knew I was amongst many powerful people, many of whom professed healing abilities in some way, so I decided I would let them come to me.

I happened to mention to someone that I wanted to stay out of my wheelchair for a few days to let this happen. Word got around and became skewed, like I was refusing to ever use my wheelchair again. The next morning, six bare-chested Israeli men appeared and said they understood why I didn't want to get in my wheelchair and insisted on carrying me. I told them that I really didn't want to be carried. These ex-soldiers would not take no for an answer and lifted me onto a cushioned bamboo platform they had built. They were in perfect step as they beared me on their shoulders from dusk till midnight for the rest of the gathering. As we walked, the sound of around forty drums beat softly seemingly in rhythm with my own heart. The whole experience had become surreal.

To some I appeared as a guru, so I blessed them with a stick. To others, a beggar, so I humbly accepted their offerings. And again, there were some who knew me and waved or ran because they knew I would be getting them to pick up rubbish or do something.

I always felt my adrenaline pumping as we headed towards the main circle. Dozens of tepees, tents and different types of camps lined our path. Each one alive with activity, some working the land, others doing workshops, all offering free food and drink. I watched people from every walk of life mingle, work and play around me as my platform swayed lightly.

I enjoyed the workshops and various gatherings with all of its curious characters and presented my own workshop in our full-sized community hall on singing affirmations. The old wooden building actually swayed slightly on its foundations as all the people sitting down inside rocked gently. I had written a song during the gathering and pinned it on the community noticeboard. As I was carried, a couple of times I could hear it being sung in more than one camp at the same time.

The night before my 30th birthday, I decided to sleep in my favourite camping spot on the property, alone. Even though there were thousands of people scattered around the land, there were still moments of absolute silence, and I fell into a deep, peaceful sleep. On awakening, I found that about 400 people had gathered at my camp to have breakfast with me for my birthday. A contingent of around forty Israeli people took control of the breakfast preparation.

It was interesting to see that the men were actually doing all the cooking. They even made sweets and fed the whole crowd. When breakfast was finished, I was asked if I would speak. People wanted to hear about my life and perspectives. A lounge chair was set up for me in the paddock next to my camp. I shared my story with everybody and a few jokes. I had been speaking for around twenty minutes when I noticed my family approaching in the distance. They seemed to have stopped and were just staring. I yelled out, 'Hey Mum!' and with that, the crowd began to naturally disperse and allow my family to come to me. My mum told me that when they saw me, they were astounded and thought they may be obliged to pray to me! That was until I yelled out and they realised it was just the same old me.

No media were allowed during the gathering, though the reports on the news from Sydney and the Gold Coast after the gathering had ended were that this healthy hippy festival had sold out the local Mount Molloy shop of all its chocolate and the Mount Carbine pub of all its beer.

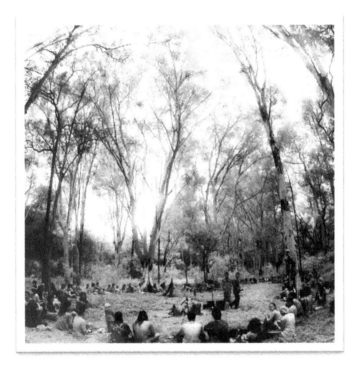

A workshop in the scrub near the main circle of Australia's first Rainbow Gathering

Around 10,000 people had attended the gathering by its end. After the gathering, a couple of dozen people wanted to stay on and became part of our community. This Rainbow Gathering brought to the surface my instinctual tribalism. It highlighted the human need to feel connected to the earth and each other, naturally.

Off-the-Grid Treasures

I had many beautiful experiences that could only come from living in a small community with a focus on self-sufficiency. Sometimes a young family, struggling with modern life or parenting, would come to stay and gain great knowledge and strength from the experience of others. It was a true treasure to see more experienced parents subtly share new or better ways with everything from tying knots to parenting, without belittling a new family in any way. Or like when a wise child, even though sometimes they were younger, would lead the new children with their love and knowledge of nature, as though they were an enchanting Pied Piper. It seemed a contrast to a normal society where people were bullied or humiliated if they were somehow different or not as knowledgeable.

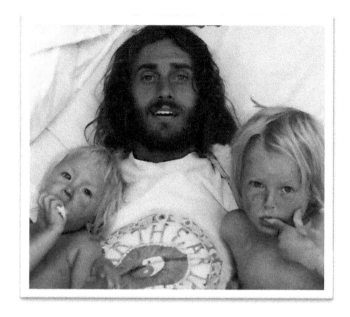

The mushroom flower children and my random Jesus look.

I remember when a small child with large, bulging blue eyes asked me if I had eaten the mushroom flowers. I was alarmed that he may have already eaten this unbeknown-to-me flower, but he beckoned me to follow him, so I did. We came to some long grass where he pointed out a weed that Jack Fisher had told me was named Bluetop.

I knew Bluetop as a natural poultice for drawing out infections in a wound. I had never noticed, but along the side of the stems were minuscule lilac flowers. The young boy picked about a dozen and gently put them in my hand. I cautiously tasted them. To my delight, they were sweet and yet had a mushroom flavour. He enquired again whether they were good to eat or not. I told him that I could not tell him any more until I investigated them further and would possibly be able to give an answer within a few hours. In fact, I was researching them and waiting to see if they poisoned me or made me hallucinate, which thank goodness for him and me, they did not.

There were many regular belly laughs about what the children were doing. One day we saw them pretending to be zebras and giraffes with their hands behind their backs, bending over and chomping on the sweet leaf. I thought, *Oh well, less lunch has to be made today!*

A few of the longer-term females approached me at a particular time with a concern. They said that after being at the sanctuary for years now and having transitioned (according to their metabolisms and constitutions) to go from vegetarians to raw foodists and then to fruitarians, they were all not having menstrual cycles and hadn't had for many months. They were worried that it had to do with their diets and could affect their ability to have children. Alarmed, I consulted books and experts only to find that in fact, it was the pain and bleeding during menstrual cycles that are normally associated with diets of cooked food that was actually unnatural. Those women continued to stay free of pain and bleeding and went on to have healthy children. Of course if you are concerned about anything that could be a serious health problem, you should always seek professional medical advice.

Having lived with a number of teenagers over the years during my time at the sanctuary, I asked myself the question that if we have evolved from Neanderthals, it would have then made sense that the strongest caveman would have had a large harem of women. That is because he would have been able to provide the greatest protection, the most food and the strongest seed for children.

Natural instinct would have been to protect the whole tribe from outsiders, who were different, thus creating bullying by natural selection. Then as the children of the tribe reached childbearing age, another natural instinct would have emerged. That being the fear of mental and physical incest, the latter resulting in genetic mutation. They, therefore, need to leave their own tribe to breed with another to keep their genes strong. Helping your 15-year-old child to understand their natural instincts could save a lot of drama.

One of Lucy's friends, Kelli, had a huge heart and was always full of positive energy. She had the idea of starting an acrobatic circus troupe for the local First Nations children. I was happy to financially sponsor the idea, and she bought things like gymnastic mats and vaults that she took wherever she went, including local Christian missions. I was watching them perform one day and decided to visit backstage. One of the young performers noticed me and innocently believing that I was a fellow performer, nonchalantly asked if my routine was a wheelchair stand. I popped it up on the back wheels for him and he said, 'I thought so' as though seeing a quadriplegic do a wheelie was a normal thing for him. The Blackrobats went on to become a highly regarded group of entertainers, travelling the world and winning international awards.

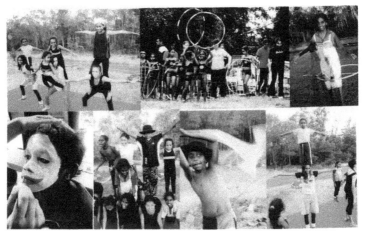

Blackrobats

From Little Things Big Things Grow

The Blackrobats of Kuranda

Having made friends when I was younger with a man named Nat through the local spiritual centre, we visited each other often. One day I learned that Nat had become acquainted with a lady named Sofi, the grandmother of the Celtic Romani Gypsies of Australia. He introduced me to her, and she told me that she was a witch. She showed me spell books handed down through the generations that contained hand-written spells and beautifully illustrated Celtic symbols.

Nat was a strong-looking, handsome young man, and Sofi was much older and embodied the characteristics of a classic-looking witch. Her love potions were well-known, and they eventually married and moved to their own property around an hour's drive away from the sanctuary. There, they grew herbs for Sofi's practice and also bush tucker trees while Sofi practised magic and Nat built websites. I had had the crazy idea of connecting the sanctuary to the neighbouring rainforest of state forest, by means of planting bush tucker trees as a corridor. I asked Nat and Sofi if I could buy some of their trees and arranged a time for them to deliver the trees to the sanctuary.

On the same day that Nat and Sofi were dropping off the trees, some of the people who lived at the sanctuary told me that there was a particular man on the property who was harassing girls. I said that we were a spiritual community and surely we could counsel him. They told me they had tried to counsel him and reason with him but it had failed, and I should ask him to leave. They then showed me a letter that he had written to one of the girls, and I realised he was sexually harassing her. I agreed that he should be asked to leave but it shouldn't be me that does it because I would interrogate him and make him confess, at which point I would most likely become angry. They disagreed and said it should come from me.

I confronted him, and he denied the accusations. I then probed him until he unintentionally spilled the beans. It did make me angry, and I asked him to leave. He became contentious so I asked some men to help him round up his stuff and escort him from the sanctuary. As they attempted to do the same, he became aggressive and loud. Just then, a person had brought me a message that Nat and Sofi, who had been enjoying a few hours at the sanctuary, were ready to leave and wanted to say goodbye. With that, I left the scene and met them in my cottage to thank them for the trees and wish them a safe journey home. Sofi had never done this before but asked me if there were any spells I would like her to do before she went. I muttered there was somebody at the sanctuary who was being a jackass. Sofi stopped me from saying anything further, especially his name. She said that she would do a general cleansing spell and that anybody whose energy was going against the community as a whole would have that same force come back at them.

Sofi asked me for a bowl. She placed it on my wooden kitchen table. In it, she placed some herbs with a clear quartz crystal on top. With a small crowd gathered around, she waved her hand over the top and said some quiet words, so as to not have people know what she said. The crystal cracked, making a horrible piercing noise. The onlookers and I were stunned. At seemingly the same moment, I heard loud yelling from the community hall. Not considering any relationship to the spell, I decided it was my duty to investigate. The jackass, in all of his wisdom, had kicked the frame of a door and subsequently broken his ankle. He had to be taken to hospital, so we threw his belongings in for the journey. Indeed, his angry energy had been returned to him.

My Friends are Frogs

Apart from learning how to manage a farm organically, we learned many techniques to do with self-sufficiency and bush crafts while living at the sanctuary. There were people who even knew how to run a car engine on water. Back then, such technology was hidden or suppressed, for fear of big companies threatening people in more ways than one. I also learned how to fix a blown light bulb by connecting it to a car battery and slowly turning the bulb until the broken filament touched and therefore fused back together because of the current.

One of the projects that we undertook as a community was to somehow get water from our all-year-round river up the embankment and to the gardens and orchards without the need for an electrical or fuel pump. After many attempts, what is known as a ram pump was built. It was a large pipe with its stainless-steel mesh-covered head pointing up to the river. Inside the pipe were a series of rubber flaps that built pressure up within each chamber. Using the right equation of length and slow undulation up the riverbank, we were successfully able to get the water to our land. This sort of system also allows the water to drop down onto a waterwheel connected to a generator that could produce electricity.

Living in just the right-sized small community, people were genuine and compassionate. Though there were times that I paid people for my care, more often people would volunteer to care for me spontaneously out of the goodness of their hearts and because they were just happy to be able to stay on the property and live a natural and fulfilling lifestyle. Regularly I would have two carers at a time doing eight hours shifts over the whole twenty-four hours of the day. Though these people were not getting paid, they were helping me with everything from exercises and getting up in the morning, to meal preparation, cleaning and being on duty overnight just in case I couldn't sleep, wanted to go for a walk, have a cup of tea or shower. I find it hard to express how humbled and appreciative this made me feel. To have that sort of support within your community is a genuine privilege, and I will never forget it.

The sanctuary developed many 'guidelines' over time, which included things such as:

- This is a place for growing, so please continue, however slowly, to transition to more spiritual, healthy and environmentally friendly lifestyles.
- Music has its appropriate times and places. Some people have come here for the music of nature.

- Please avoid bringing any animal products or toxic substances like inorganic fertilisers, chemicals, metals not part of a healthy body, and other unnatural substances.
- Please keep all things clean and hygienic, and if you can, even better than the way you found it.

Smoking, alcohol and drugs were discouraged. We found that the body had many natural drugs more powerful than anything that is external or can be synthesised. Adrenaline, dopamine, endorphins and the power found in our pituitary and pineal glands could be activated internally and induce a state of bliss and high awareness when needed.

Eventually, I decided to stop random tourists from being able to drive through or around our sanctuary and camp or swim above us in the river. This was because of the amount of rubbish I would find, next to or in the river, including disposable nappies and empty toothpaste, soap and shampoo containers.

One day we had some students and professors from a nearby university camp on our property and the surrounding area for a couple of weeks while they studied the environment. They came to me towards the end of their stay and were talking to me about their findings when they opened up a poster with brightly coloured photos of six of Queensland's missing frogs. They then said something that was to become one of the greatest treasures of my soul in life. Maybe my proudest moment. It both rewarded and emboldened my spirit. They meekly announced that during their time there, they had now found four of these extinct frogs, within my sanctuary.

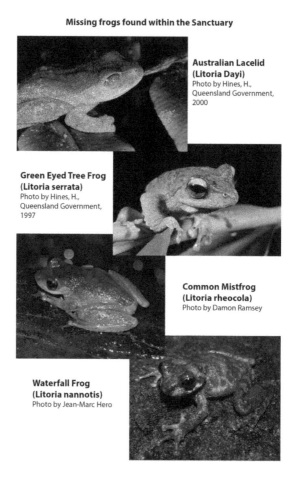

Missing frogs found within the Sanctuary

Australian Lacelid (Litoria Dayi)
Photo by Hines, H., Queensland Government, 2000

Green Eyed Tree Frog (Litoria serrata)
Photo by Hines, H., Queensland Government, 1997

Common Mistfrog (Litoria rheocola)
Photo by Damon Ramsey

Waterfall Frog (Litoria nannotis)
Photo by Jean-Marc Hero

I never knew what it was that I was actually trying to achieve in my life, and especially at the sanctuary, until that moment. Now I knew I had created a true sanctuary. I knew that frogs were vital to keeping our rivers and waterways clean and without them, we wouldn't be able to drink the water. A warm rush and titillating buzz travelled from the tip of my feet to the top of my head.

We had spent much time protecting the river from tourists, fighting fires and rehabilitating the riverbanks with vegetation, so I felt a great sense of satisfaction and achievement of my goals.

I really felt like I was a true gatekeeper of paradise.

Tie His Schlong to His Leg

After my out-of-court settlement, I honestly believed that I would never run out of money. But a mere five years later, after dishing out over a half a million dollars to my immediate family, giving ten or twenty thousand dollars to another dozen people or so, carers wages, paying my legal team and paying back social security, along with the purchase of my property and some vehicles, I was beginning to run low.

To me, the sanctuary had always been more of a refuge for wildlife and for people needing a home or healing than a place of business. Its focus was never to try to aggressively make money, yet we knew it had to continue to financially sustain itself. So, over time we developed business ideas and took ways to make money a little more importantly.

The sanctuary was getting busy and with plenty of W.W.O.O.Fers arriving, we were preparing our products for market, which included fresh fruit, dried fruit, honey from our hives and tree seedlings. One of the tree seedlings was Neem, which we were selling a local council to plant and thus keep down the population of sandflies and mosquitos.

Tourists and locals alike would scratch themselves after being bitten, and the bite often turned into a tropical ulcer. Neem was a strategy to reduce hospital visits and seemed to work. Other sources of income included a small weekly fee for rent for people who didn't want to do the four hours of work per week together as a community (unless a person had no income and was physically unable at the same time) along with money from our donation box and honesty box from our stall outside our front gate. We were also attending to a constant demand for our Lotus flower products from florists and little old ladies, along with managing a growing interest in the leasing of areas for animal agistment.

The mango season was approaching as well, which meant there was lots of picking, packing and delivering to do. I decided to look for hired help in management. I found a man living at the sanctuary who was suitable for the job. He was older than me and had the right qualifications. I said that he could handpick a team of men from the sanctuary to assist him in his duties, and knowing the nature of the men, I was sure they would be happy to volunteer their time, to which they did. He was doing a good job with everything running smoothly, and I felt some pressure lift from my shoulders.

A few weeks later he approached me with his group of men. They had a worried look on their faces and told me they needed to speak with me about something. Concerned that it was something serious, I immediately gave them my attention.

'We need to do something about the 'Frenchman'. He is walking around naked and getting all the girls. He has a big shlong.'

I looked at them and laughed. They were not laughing! 'What? You are kidding, right?' I said.

'No, we're not. We need to do something about it.'

I knew that there were a lot of people walking around naked. It was obvious to me that the 'Frenchman', who was supposedly getting all the girls, was not getting them only because of his shlong. These guys were mostly meat-eating, alcohol-drinking, cigarette-smoking, bone-headed yobbos. Most of the girls on the other hand, were sensitive, health-focused, fairy-type beings. They had no chance in hell of seducing one of these girls.

'Aaah, do you notice that the Frenchman makes the girls breakfast in the mornings, offers them massages, is the first to get the firewood each day and plays beautiful songs to the girls on his guitar? Should I make a rule just for the Frenchman? The Frenchman must tie his shlong to his leg? Go away,' I said.

They were very upset that I did not take their problem seriously as they turned with their heads hung and walked away.

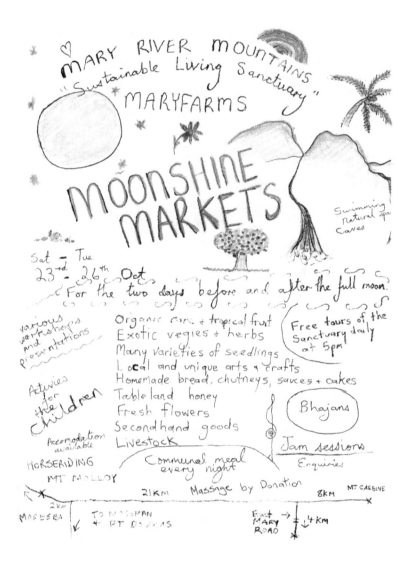

The sanctuary full moon markets, held outside of our front gates. Since my injury, my hands are not fully functional so I drew this with my mouth.

Backwards Walked the
Black Witch

Not everything is always perfect in paradise. Most rural prop-
erties in Australia are laid back and security is not an issue.
Universal law though, is that if you do not secure something,
you may lose it. Australian law is similar. Our law states that if
you leave your property open, whether it's the door on your
unit or the farm fence gate, it is an open invitation for people
to enter. A piece of string across an entrance is classed as being secure but an open gate or door is not. If someone enters
and you do not have a verbal or written agreement with them,
they can squat, mark out an area and make a claim with the
Department of Natural Resources. This is basic squatters'
rights. If the door or gate is closed and they open it, they are
trespassing.

Having invited a friend, known by the name of Carlita, to come and stay at the sanctuary some time back, I arrived home one day to find her there. She had set up a camp with her whole tribe, which at the time I was fine with. What I thought might be a stay of days had turned to weeks and then to months. Now Carlita knew our system was that people who were staying any longer than one week did a half of a day's work with the community once a week or paid $40. Despite this, Carlita's tribe would neither work with us nor pay. It soon became apparent that in fact, they were working against us. When we were using irrigation at one end of the property, they would be using it at the other, rendering the pressure in both areas of almost no use. Some would speed through the property in their vehicle and have no regard for the children's safety. Enough was enough, and people began to complain about them.

Several appeals to them for fairness failed to change anything. Eventually, the decision was made to ask them to leave. They bluntly refused and dialogue continued on the matter for many weeks. During one confrontation that I had with Carlita and her tribe, another resident approached with news of a mutual friend being hurt in a car crash. Carlita immediately took credit for the hurting of our friend, stating that our friend had done something to her (which was menial), so she had cast a spell on them. I was taken aback, considering this to be black witchcraft.

That was it, no more talk. It was time to get heavy. I gathered a troop of strong men that were prepared to physically escort them from the premises. We arrived to find they had barricaded themselves with razor wire! They then appeared with guns! We did not have guns and did not want a gun fight.

I called the police. When they arrived, they asked me if I had a written or verbal agreement with them. I told the police that I had said to them that they could come and stay. The police told me that was a verbal agreement and that it was open-ended. The police then asked how Carlita had entered the property. I said that the gate is always open. The police then told me that leaving the gate open is a free invitation for the public to enter anytime and they could claim squatter's rights. They said there was nothing the police could do.

I clenched my jaw and did circles in my wheelchair. I felt as though there was some sort of spell over me or the sanctuary. If she was a black witch, she may have used a curse. I decided there was one last thing that I would try. I would call on my own magic powers.

I began to fast. I would chant and visualise the positive outcome I was seeking. I did not sleep. I remained in the lotus position. I sweated and my body shook. A concerned friend slept at my feet. I conversed with gods and could hear the witch's incantations.

On the fourth night, just before dawn, a bright and beautiful light appeared before me. It was welcoming and enticing. I decided that I was fed up with this world and I would go into the light. The only way I could do that was if I was willing to leave everything in this world behind. One by one, I let go of all things. Firstly, my material possessions, which also meant the sanctuary. Then my friends, family and loved ones. Finally, there was only my body to let go of, and my spirit would fly free to the light. Suddenly, I felt a weight lift, and I remembered what had brought me to where I was. Because I had no attachment to the world now at this point, it had no power over me. Therefore, along with that, any spell or curse of any witch. I realised that I had achieved what it was I was trying to do regarding the witch. That morning, Carlita and her tribe were seen walking backwards out of the property, never to return. These days, we are best friends again, and it is a testament to our renewed friendship that she allowed me to include this story about our past.

Scratching My Neck

Every year the farmers in the area would get together to do some back burning to ensure the whole community of Maryfarms was safe from bush fires. The bush fire season lasted for about four months. Each year another farmer would take their turn as fire chief. This year it was my turn. The fire chief was responsible for central co-ordination and most importantly having extra fuel on hand for any generators that were being used to fight a particular fire so that it didn't become out of control. Equally as important was his job as supplier of the beer at the end of the day.

We decided to start the burning around the borders of my farm, as it was the last property before the mountains, and work our way back to the highway. People and all types of vehicles from every farm in the region began to arrive. A semi-trailer tanker of water, bulldozers, graders and tractors pulled in. Most were a ute with a trailer that had a water tank, a generator, a fire hose and a mob of very hick-looking volunteers. Weather and equipment were checked, and roads were readied. A match was lit and the danger began.

I listened intensely to the advice and instructions of the older and more experienced farmers. There was a lot of yelling about checking the intensity of particular fires and making sure people were not burning themselves or anybody else into a corner. Embers were being chased into the bush and extinguished most thoroughly. About halfway through the day, things were running semi-smoothly. We had, however, used more emergency fuel than expected, so I told one of the elder men I needed to organise more fuel and asked if he would take the reins.

I returned with the fuel and enough beer for everybody. At the end of the day, everybody was relieved that there were no major incidences, and we were safe from fires for another year. I leaned with my elbow on the extremely large esky of beer. I looked around to see many dry mouths. There were blackened faces and many tall hats. Cane farmers, cow cockies, hippies and even squatters had all gathered for their beer reward. I couldn't help myself. This was a classic opportunity.

I yelled out, 'Aye, what's a redneck?'

Everyone turned and looked at me. Some had suddenly looked like they were ready to lynch me. After an awkward pause, I said, 'A redneck is a young city slicker who comes to the bush and thinks he knows everything but after a while he finds himself scratching his neck, thinking I should have just asked my neighbours for help years ago!'

For some reason, there were only a couple of laughs. I quickly opened the esky.

Voicing Peace of Mind

Some days I liked to just enjoy parts of the sanctuary by myself and would look for places flat enough that I could push my wheelchair without the need of anybody's help. It was one such day when I was near the end of the property that one of the squatters from the adjacent land came to talk with me. Unlike some of the other squatters we would find sometimes trying to steal tools or fruit, Justin was a good man. He regularly offered free help to the community and kept a very functional campsite. His veggie patch was always abundant, and the drains around his tent were well maintained. Justin was also a mathematical genius. He could make equations that tiered out both sides like a flower in bloom.

Justin looked slightly troubled this day, and I asked him if everything was okay. He told me that years ago he had been diagnosed with schizophrenia. He said that he had tried many techniques and medications to no avail. Although he had lived in the bush now for years, Justin said that the voices in his head were still so loud, it was like a gigantic crowd having a party. I asked if he was wanting my suggestion. He laughed and said, 'Well, we are the only people for as far as the eye can see.'

I told him that something came to me instinctively. I asked him to go home and get everything done for the night so he could sit down and focus. I asked Justin what the most masculine voice was that he could imagine. I said, 'If God were a male, what would his voice sound like to you?' I then used my most masculine voice as an example. It was deep and commanding. It resonated with authority. I told him to find that voice in himself. I said for him to speak it as loud as he could in his own mind. I suggested that he use it to demand silence of all the other voices. I reasoned with him regarding his birth as a male and to use that power in all its glory. Justin accepted my challenge and said it seemed to make perfect sense. He would go away and try it.

I saw Justin the next day. He had a grin from ear to ear. He said that he had done exactly what I said and prepared himself for the night but when he first tried it, he could not hear his voice. After perseverance, he did begin to hear his voice but it was soft, in no way a voice of God and not even manly. He worked on making it louder until it became the loudest voice, eventually finding his 'voice of God'. He had commanded silence, loudly, in his mind at the crowd. And with that, they had all then fallen silent.

Unfortunately, it only lasted a moment. One by one, they were trying to come back and dominate his headspace again. Only this time, he recognised each and every one of them. They were not some random voices, spirits or aliens. And they were certainly not the multiple personalities suggested by his psychiatrist. They were the voices of his mother, a teacher, a friend, an actor and a TV ad to an ex-girlfriend, an enemy, a radio announcer and everybody in between. He silenced every one of them individually and finally found peace of mind again.

This voice has served me well both in times where a strong or quick decision was needed to be made or peace and calm were required. I have also allowed myself to hear the 'voice of the goddess', which seems to have the power of subtlety, softness, sweetness and beauty in all of its feminine glory.

What is your voice of God? Speak to yourself with this voice. Every word will have endless power. And the slower that you speak each word in your mind, the more powerful Each Single Word Will Be.

An Ocean of Emotion

Jack Fisher had been battling for a few years now with prostate cancer. In his last days, I brought him home to live with me and tried to make him comfortable. Jack passed away soon after. As he had made me the executor of his Will, I began to put his affairs in order, including trying to contact his family for the funeral. A large number of people attended Jack's funeral but unfortunately no family. Jack had also made me the only beneficiary of his Will, and after paying all of his bills, I was left with $4700.47. The number 47 was my favourite number, having popped up in my life very many times, and Jack knew that. Surely, he could not have orchestrated for my favourite number to be part of his parting gift? In years to come, I was to experience that Jack was not finished with me yet.

I intended to live out my life in the sanctuary and had never, ever contemplated sale.

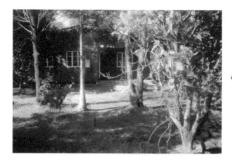

**A house located
near the river**

**A cottage at the
end of the orchid**

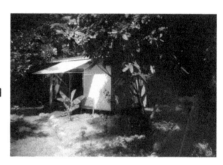

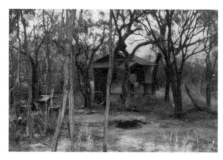

A random shack
Located in the
bush near one of
the paddocks.

Sanctuary buildings.

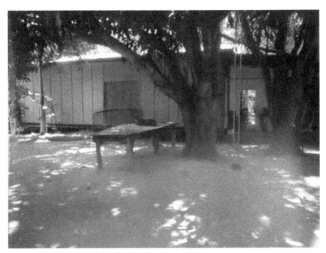

Our community hall after doing some renovations
The two mango trees on the right were 80 years old and gave
off thousands of fruits each season. Their roots reached
down into the water table of the river just 50 metres away.

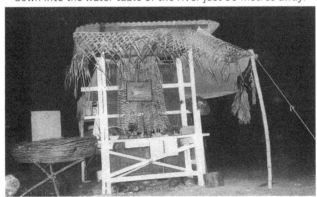

Our front gate market stall
Even though we were 4km from the main road, our honesty
box had money in it nearly every day.

Sanctuary buildings.

We lived the most ideal lifestyle, but even so it was hard at times. I had never intended to be a primary producer, and on top of that I was a quadriplegic trying to take care of a large organic, self-sufficient sanctuary. However, one day I was approached by somebody I knew with an offer to buy with plans to keep everything the same, allowing me to live there but have money to invest in the property. Unfortunately, after the sale, the new owner and I had a falling out. Not long after, they developed a serious health issue and passed away.

Losing the sanctuary in this fashion devastated me. I felt that I had lost a part of myself. The man that I originally bought the sanctuary from was hired to take over management. The strange cycle has circled, and I hope my turn will come again soon.

Trying to be Normal

I felt very lost without the sanctuary and all of its wonderful characters. Nevertheless, I had to face reality and try to be part of general society and unfortunately suburbia again. Wondering what to do next, I decided to buy a house in Smithfield Heights. The property had a great work shed, and I could see the ocean from my backyard.

I began renovating away. I changed ceilings, walls, floors and nearly everything in between for a year and a half. During that time, I went to Melbourne and did some hyperbaric oxygen chamber therapy for six weeks at a cost of $600 per day. It did yield some slight improvements but not enough to justify its continuation. I have tried many other things over the years and will continue to, though as time passes, scarring and atrophy of the spinal cord does make it harder for any healing techniques to work. In saying that, for people with newly acquired spinal cord injuries, there are wonderful new scientific discoveries and techniques that are indeed helping people all over the world now.

I took my trusty friend and carer of the same name as my former friend, Jack Fisher, with me to Melbourne. This new Jack Fisher I had met at the sanctuary. He had arrived with another man that he was working for, just to earn his keep. I noticed that he was personable and a great worker. As I got to know him more, I understood that he had much wisdom, always dressed well and even smelled good! I'd convinced him to stay with me at the sanctuary and he became loved by all. When I eventually sold, he had still been living there. Subsequently, I told him he could come wherever I went. This second Jack Fisher in my life became a great friend, living with me in the next few places on my journeys. We are still close to this day.

Back then my injury and circumstances began to get to me. I started to use painkillers, which soon became the abuse of them. Within no time at all, I was a junkie.

I broke my painkillers down to inject them by needle two or three times a day.

No words can describe the desperation a person feels with a heavy addiction. My mind was weak, and my body was caught in a vicious cycle. If I did not get my fix on time, I would begin to become anxious, nauseous, shaking and sweating with my heart beating so hard I could feel it nearly pumping out of my chest.

I decided I had endured enough in this lifetime and would finally end it all by taking my life. Over the course of the next year-and-a-half, I tried to either give away or spend all my money, while I tried to write my life story. I sold my house and moved to a five-star hotel for six months, hiring six secretaries. The wild sex must have distracted me, so I rented a mansion instead. Another year became a grey haze before I started to see that despite my wanton destruction, people still loved me, and I still loved a lot of people and life itself. I began to perceive a glimpse of hope in the future and decided it was better to continue to live, no matter how hard it might be. I slowly weened myself from the drugs. After many attempts, I was clean again. Never could I have imagined that I would allow emotions to control me so much or a physical substance to threaten my life.

Having spent or given away all my money, and ten years after my settlement, I was on the bones of my arse again. I made the decision to go back into the workforce. Because I felt I had to start in the lowliest of places, I began to study for my Real Estate Licence. I got the first job I applied for and commenced my cheesy sales career. My first listing was a two-storey house. I wondered how I would show people upstairs. At the same time, I had been looking for a new carer. My friend Jed had met a young fellow while hitchhiking whom he relayed the same to.

The young fellow told Jed that his girlfriend was looking for a job, and Jed told me. He told me that her name was Katie but that she was only seventeen. I said, 'No way! She will have no brains, be always taking drugs and want every weekend off!'

Jed brought her around to my place anyway. I looked her up and down and tried to be tough. She said, 'I have always wanted to become a nurse and if I got this job, I would study to become a nurse.'

Damn it! I thought. *She wants to be a nurse. Awwww, s**t, f**k, I am an a**hole if I don't give her a job.* I gave Katie a go. I told her she had to help me sell the two-storey house on the weekend. She turned up with a very short skirt and low top and the house sold immediately.

Katie applied to study at TAFE, and I wrote a letter commending her. They offered her a $6500 grant and she became an enrolled nurse. She went on to become a registered nurse and is now the head of her ward at the hospital. Katie is my longest-serving carer and is like a daughter to me. When I told her she was in my Will, she told me she would marry me for the last year of my life so that she could get everything. I thought about it and then realised the only way she could know that it was my last year was if she planned to kill me! Haha. She is now married (not to me thank goodness), has bought her first home and recently gave birth to two wonderful twin boys.

One day Katie was helping me get dressed when she said, 'I think I have been working with you long enough now that I can tell you your balls are starting to droop.'

'You cheeky bugger!' I said. 'You are a nurse now so you can stitch them back up, hey bitch?' Katie's cheek continues to add spice to my life and keeps me on my toes (or air in my tyres).

I once had a girlfriend do some care shifts with me. Some shifts were quite party-like with wild sex, drinking, smoking and forgetting to do my exercises. One time she helped me get into my shower chair after such a shift and I became light-headed, fainting and falling forward into her bare breasts. She didn't realise I was unconscious and thought I was nuzzling her breasts. Jed happened to walk past and caught a glimpse of us through the open door. He saw my face was blue. He quickly came in and sat me up, slapped me about and got me breathing again. Although it was traumatic, I have decided that it is the way I would like to die. And as for Jed saving my life, I think that it stands at five times now.

Around the same time one of my wonderful carers, Emma, and her sweet little daughter, Jordyn, had a wonderful rapport with her border collie dog. It was intelligent, obedient and fun. I hadn't owned a dog since I was a boy and considered whether it could be a good thing for me. I decided it was, and that a border collie would suit me well. I soon found a beautiful puppy that I named Bowie. Katie and I then began the long process of training him to the licensed level of an Assistance Dog. It was a wonderful experience and one that we would do several times over a dozen years, including for other people.

The Crazy With Pink Earrings

My great niece Lizzie, my carer Katie and I all decided to go for a walk one morning to the local shops, across from a house I was renting down in town. We finished our business there and had one last thing to do, which was to pick up a bottle of Jack Daniels as a birthday gift for a friend of mine. In those days Katie still smoked cigarettes, so we waited by the notice board out the front of the liquor store for her to finish her smoke. Two young men entered the liquor store, and I heard Katie take a deep breath and sigh. I asked her if everything was okay. She told me that the two young men we had just seen owed her money from the sale of one of her puppies but had still not paid after months.

I was immediately angered as Katie worked hard for her money, caring for such a hard case like me. Apart from that, the puppy was part of a litter from another puppy that I had given to Katie years ago. She had spent much time and money on all the worming and immunisation required for new puppies. I told her to finish her smoke and that I would get the Jack Daniels myself. She knew what I was up to and only half-heartedly tried to stop me because she really wanted me to do something and knew deep down that she had no chance of stopping me.

I entered the liquor store and shuffled the bottle onto my lap. The two young men were already in line at the counter with only one person in front of them. I headed towards the counter and aggressively pushed in front of them. I purposely knocked them with my wheelchair, and they looked away as though I was obviously just a disgruntled person in a wheelchair or maybe a person who had mental health issues. The two old ladies at the counter politely helped me with my wallet and to finish my transaction. I thanked them and smiled.

I then swung around wildly, smashing into the young men's legs and bottles. I told them that I knew that they owed Katie money, which now meant that they owed me money. I relayed how that Katie worked hard for her money because I was an a**hole. I assured them that if they did not pay, I would not be so nice next time. With their mouths opened wide, they nodded and agreed to pay. They must have thought that if a quadriplegic was threatening them, he must have either the means to do what he says or is just bats**t crazy. Either way, it was probably better just to do what he said. I turned again to thank the old ladies at the counter one more time. They were horrified and were happy to see me leave.

When we got home, I happened to pass by a mirror when I saw the pink sticker earrings that I had forgotten Lizzie had put on me before we left. Katie had her money within a week.

The Phoenix Jack

One day a young lady was sent to me through a care service, named Helen. Unlike many I had encountered, she was sweet. After about six weeks of working together, she arrived for one of her regular shifts. I asked how she was and then asked a question that I would not usually ask. For some reason, I asked what she was doing after work. Normally, I would not ask personal questions. She told me that her boyfriend and her had decided that today they would look for where his grandfather was laid to rest as nobody in the family knew where it was. Intrigued, I enquired about the grandfather. As she spoke of him, his delightful character and colourful life, I had a warm wind blow over the entirety of my body. I realised that I was the only person in the whole world who knew the answer to the question of where he was laid to rest. It was Jack Fisher.

It had been six years since the passing of my great friend Jack Fisher, but he obviously hadn't gone too far. After the settlement for my injury, I had given Jack money. And though he was estranged from his family, he had visited his son and used the money to buy his grandson a motorbike. I told Helen who I was. She burst into tears. She then thanked me for the motorbike, which started my waterworks. We agreed that Jack had been guiding our every step to bring us together on that particular day, probably even whispering that unusual question in my ear. Jack had unfinished business with his family and could not rest until he could finally reach his grandson. I feel honoured to have been the vessel to do so. I was able to take Helen and Jack's grandson, Shane, to where I had spread Jack's ashes and share with them all of his wisdom and adventures.

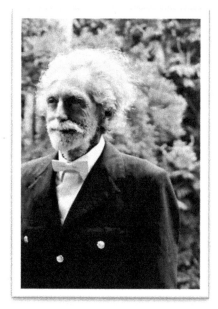

The fantastic Jack Fisher. It was like having a mystical wizard as a mentor. A friend in deed and in spirit

The Night Job

Joan had been sent to care for me by one of the bigger services in town. I came to know her more and more over the few months she had been working with me and she seemed like a fairly normal, quiet type of person. I had decided that I needed more care hours than what I was getting and would employ an extra full-time person from my own money. I knew that Joan was unhappy with her employer and they were not giving her as many hours as she would have liked, so I offered her the position. We agreed to a starting date for her, around a week before Xmas. Though I was now in my early thirties and lived by myself, my mum was a regular visitor and made Joan promise she would take care of me, especially over the Xmas period while Mum was away on holidays.

The day came for Joan to start full-time, but she was late. After a while, I became concerned and tried to ring. There was no answer. I left it a while longer and sent a text, still with no reply. When an hour or more had passed, my thoughts were becoming worrying. Has she slept through an alarm? Is she ill? Has she been arrested for something? Was she in an accident?

Having met her brother, whom Joan lived with along with her partner, I remembered that I had her brother's phone number as well. I rang him and told him that Joan had not turned up for work. He sounded puzzled, stating that it was strange that she was supposed to be working because she had left for Adelaide a few days beforehand and was not due back until the new year. I was mystified of course, along with being angry that she had for some reason not even bothered to tell me she wouldn't be turning up. Lucky my faithful friend Jed stepped straight in to care for me until I could find a replacement.

Two weeks after New Year, Joan decided to send a text announcing that she would start work the next week. I could not believe the gall. My reply was to remind her that the job was supposed to start a month ago and therefore I had already hired someone else. Joan erupted in a flurry of abusive texts. She accused me of ruining her life. Of course, I took no notice of her anger and politely said goodbye.

Around two weeks later, I was up late doing maintenance on my computer. Those were the days when one needed to perform a manual defragmentation to keep the machine from slowing down. I unplugged the phone cord to the Internet and began the long, arduous process. I finished around 2 a.m., turned off the lamp and fell into a deep sleep. Soon after, I woke to the sound of my bedroom door opening internally from the lounge room. I knew that I was supposed to be the only one home. My heart pounded.

The light from the lounge area had been switched on, and I saw the silhouette of a man rush towards me. He was wearing a balaclava and held what appeared to be a crowbar above my head, in a threatening shake. 'Where is your bag?' he asked aggressively.

Where is my bag? I thought. Only somebody that knew me, or knew about me, would ask such a question. Otherwise, they would have asked where my money or wallet was. This made me angry. I knew that I had a bag with old paperwork behind my door and that it had a lock on it. I also knew that I had a mate who was a security guard. He lived a few hundred metres away and another at about the same distance who was a martial arts expert. I surmised that I would direct him to the useless bag, and he would take it and go, only realising it wasn't the bag he was after when he finally broke it open. Surely this would give me five or ten minutes, in which time I would ring my friends with my mobile and they would come to my aid.

Sure enough, he took the bait and went. Very pleased with myself but still in shock with adrenaline pumping, I sat up my electric bed, turned on the touch lamp and reached for my mobile. It was gone. Evidently, the crook had been in my bedroom beforehand, relieved me of my only means of communication and not found the bag. I knew this meant that when he came back, as he surely would, he would be angrier and possibly violent.

With the Internet unplugged and the phone line on the floor, I could not even contact any friend who might happen to be online at that ungodly hour. A very tense and frightening few minutes passed. Suddenly he appeared and ran toward me. He was very angry and with the crowbar raised high he bellowed, 'We have a problem!'

He wasn't wearing his balaclava, and I had the lamp still turned on, so this time there was no hiding his from face me. I did not recognise him but made sure I looked at him long and hard before I decided to answer him.

'So, you must mean the bag with my money in it, hey mate?' I said angrily.

I detected a slight look of guilt on his face, so I played it. 'Actually buddy, I'm over having this disability and I'm over people like you. I have been waiting for a weak piece of crap like you to come along, so go ahead and kill me, I am ready to die, just make sure you do actually kill me, because if you don't, I will come after you and you will suffer a worse fate than me, and jail after that. I know your face now and because you asked for my bag, not my money or wallet, I know this is an inside job and it's not hard to guess who has sent you. So, tell Joan I will be coming for her as well.'

My guess was right. His jaw dropped, and he lowered the crowbar. 'I'm sorry, mate. I'm a speed addict and I owe money. If I don't take your bag to her, she said she will cut off my supply and have me beaten up.'

After everything that had happened, it did not surprise me that Joan was a drug dealer. I thought to myself, *If this guy has a*

bad enough addiction to break into a house and steal from a disabled
person, he is still likely to attack me or vandalise my home if I do not give
him my bag.

'Okay then, how about you leave my bag and just take the money?' I asked.

He answered, 'She told me I have to take the bag.'

'Alright, take the bag and the money but please leave my identification and cards,' I pleaded.

He agreed, and I told him where the bag was. He asked me as he was leaving if I would like him to try to fix the door that he had unhinged. I probably could have asked him to make me a cup of tea at that point and he would have said yes.

I said, 'No, just go please.' And with that, he left.

I thought about the rest of the things in my house that he had left behind. Large screen TVs, laptops and jewellery. Concerned that he or one of his friends could yet return again, I decided I needed to contact someone. Using the electric bed remote control, I managed to hook the phone line up from the floor and eventually was able to plug it back into the computer. None of my friends were online and to my amazement, I discovered that all emergency services in Australia are not contactable over the Internet and there is not even a chat facility for them. If you needed to quietly contact emergency services, you would think that the Internet would be the best way. Unfortunately, it remains the same to this day.

I racked my brain and decided the best idea to find somebody awake online at the hour would be to join a dating site. The first person who talked to me was a male. Yes, I am so pretty he must have thought I was a girl. I told him my dilemma and asked him to ring the police. Unfortunately, he was in the United Arab Emirates and his mobile phone would not allow him to ring our emergency number.

Thankfully, a lady from Rockhampton decided to chat with me. When I asked her if she would ring the police for me, she hesitated. I decided to ask her to ring my mum instead. She agreed. I said to her to tell my mum not to come herself but to send the police. Mum arrived minutes later accompanied by a very old man that could hardly walk. I was angry that she had turned up before the police but gladder to see her.

I stewed on my injustice and decided that the police would be too slow to act and possibly not be able to prove the crime or find enough evidence to convict Joan. I felt as though I would not sleep properly the next night unless I did something. I contacted my friend who advised me to wait until the next night when we had organised enough backup to confront her. I was not willing to wait. I remembered my biker friends and rang them to tell them what had happened. They said their boss would not be very happy that Joan was selling speed or with what she had done to me. They told me that they had a job already scheduled for that night, so if I could wait until another night, it would be better. I said thank you, but I needed to do this straight away. They wished me all power.

I decided I would wait until near midnight, wrap a chain around my wrist and give a visit to Joan and her boyfriend. I asked one of my carers if they would stay late that night and help me get in and out of bed. They agreed. When the time came, they helped me get into my wheelchair, and I asked them to pass me the chain. Of course, the carer questioned me, but I would not tell them what I was going to do. They declared that if I did not let them come with me that they would follow me anyway. After a fair bit of argument, I decided to tell them what I needed to do. They were adamant that they were coming with me. I said that if they did, I would sack them. They said they were willing to be sacked. After some compromise, I allowed the carer to come and sit in the pub that happened to be across the road from where Joan lived. They could only watch through the window but if for some reason I seemed to be in trouble, only then were they allowed to send somebody from the pub to help me. They agreed.

I drove into Joan's yard and saw that the light was on upstairs. I proceeded to yell, telling them to come down and face me. I began to smash everything from the letterbox to car windows and house windows. No one appeared. After about a ten or fifteen-minute rampage, I decided that the police would arrive any moment, so I meandered over to the pub and enjoyed a beer.

The next day, Joan and her boyfriend rocked up at my home. I was alarmed and ready for anything. They told me that they were sorry and were leaving town. I told them that they better had. They left town and have since tried to contact me asking for forgiveness. I don't think the bikers have forgiven them.

The Rollover of the Standover

I was on my way back up in life again after ditching the drug habit, working as a real estate agent and starting my own disability access consultancy. With itchy feet, I decided to rent a flash place with an indoor heated wheelchair-accessible pool. I was back in Kuranda, my old stomping ground. Unfortunately, I still had not learned to fully transmute or channel my anger in sudden confrontations, and I was about to be pushed to the edge.

With renewed vigour, I canvassed local businesses and pitched them my consultancy services. At one stage I had gotten into a long, friendly conversation with a local policeman about Assistance Dogs when I realised that I was in fact supposed to be at a doctor's appointment. I quickly excused myself and hurriedly set off towards town. As I rounded the corner of the top pub, I heard the voice of 'Kurt' swearing angrily about tourists. Now, Kuranda is a town whose main income is from tourism, and I recalled when I had to ban Kurt from the sanctuary after I found him stealing. I tried to ignore him and continued on my way.

Approaching the doctors, I was stunned to see my mum standing out the front of the surgery, pale and with her mouth open as though she had seen a ghost.

'Mum, what's wrong?' I said with concern.

'I've just had the worst verbal abuse in my life. You know him. It's that Kurt. I had a win on the pokies and was walking out of the pub very happy, when he called me an old s**t and then worse than that. He also abused another old lady and some young Japanese tourists. I complained to the manager, but they did nothing.'

I was enraged. Kurt was full of muscles, and I had heard he had now become a standover man, heavying people for whatever he could hustle.

I calmly attended my appointment and then headed to the pub. At top speed, I skidded sideways into the garden bar and the middle of a seated crowd. 'Where's Kurt, the big man?'

Somebody answered, 'He's in the lounge bar, with an underage girl sitting on his lap.'

I was even angrier. I turned to see him in the distance and headed straight towards him. I smashed into his legs at top speed, which propelled my body forward. I made sure my elbow landed squarely in his throat and I followed through with a well-timed head-butt. Kurt dropped and looked confused. I told him in some choice words not to abuse my mother or anybody else for that matter.

One of his group yelled out, 'I knew you couldn't get away with that, Kurt.'

Another of his mates, Jock, got to his feet, only to ask me if I needed help. I knew Jock's dad well. 'I don't need your help and you'll be next if you keep hanging around with this idiot,' I said.

Immediately the manager and a bouncer appeared. They grabbed Kurt (not me) and dragged him out while he protested. I told him that he had better leave town because I would bash him every time I saw him from now on. The manager bought me a rum, and the crowd cheered me as I rolled away. I'm not trying to inflate my ego by relaying this story; I'm rather hoping to portray the ability of the fearless and bold spirit. It's never the size of the dog in the fight, it's the size of the fight in the dog.

I have, however, come to understand that when anger turns to violence, it is unproductive and it is certainly not the real me. These days, if I feel that I really need to impart a lesson to somebody in particular, the most powerful means for me is to find the common ground or sometimes create a joke about the whole thing. These approaches can break even the tensest situation and cause people to contemplate the bigger picture or a more subtle truth at the time. They also tend to look back at such incidences and see the mistakes clearly.

Taking Care of Business

Katie was studying to be a nurse when she first started with me in 2005, and she was paid a simple government carer's pension to assist me. At the same time, I had been allocated some funding through the government for other workers to be paid through care services, like the one that Helen was sent from. I became frustrated with the restrictions and bureaucracy of the care services with their lack of transparency or access to management. I was, however, happy with Katie's management and her dedication, so I enquired of the government if I could manage the money allocated to me without the need for the care services. I was told that it could not be done. I decided to look at the relevant legislation and seemed to find that it could. I highlighted the text and sent a copy to the local department. They declared that I was right, and in 2007 I started my own company.

After a couple of years, I had mastered all the aspects of running a company: employing people, developing policies, accounting and dealing with the government. I could employ who I wanted to do whatever I wanted, whenever I wanted. My life was full; I had my privacy back and my carers seemed to be happy. I decided that I could do as good a job or better than other care services so applied to the department to be approved as a care service in my own right for other people that needed care.

Being approved by the department, I began to take on clients. I managed the service for a few years before a young fellow from Kuranda that I had known since he was just a small boy, Dylan, joined our team and took up a position as co-ordinator. He did a wonderful job, and we developed what was to become a long-term friendship. We cared for everybody from those who just wanted us to have a cup of coffee with them, to transsexual people with a disability and children with severe autism. We cared for some people 24/7, having live-in workers, and some nights found ourselves awake at midnight counselling suicidal teenagers. The work was complex, sometimes hard, but always rewarding. The team of some twenty carers were my personal heroes, sincere and devoted.

Over time I had become further frustrated with government processes and the lack of support for some people that seemed to have the greatest need. The profit we made over those years only seemed to just cover costs, and my health was suffering. Dylan was making a decent wage but I was not able to take a wage. The way funding for the care of people from the state government was distributed in those days was very restrictive. Together we decided that it was more manageable and only profitable if I went back to being the manager, with only as many clients as I could manage myself. Dylan's wife was pregnant and it was near Christmas, so I said we should push through until the new year. He was adamant that I should not allow my health to suffer. It was hard to let the clients and employees go, but we knew we had to. I took Dylan to lunch at the casino on his last shift, and he won $20,000 on the pokies. We felt the universe was once again backing us in anything we decided to do.

Within a couple of years, I went back to work full of energy and new ideas. This next time I completely messed it up.

I decided to once again provide a care service, but this time also sell mobility equipment, the cheapest medical supplies in Australia and a range of groceries at a lower cost than the major supermarkets. We opened a shop in the city and seemed to be always busy but never making enough money again.

The government gave us no help or clients, and our landlord embarked on years of renovations in our arcade. I realised I had tried to do too much at once, too cheaply. This was along with the harsh realisation that if you offer things too cheaply, Australians believe it must be an inferior product. People would rather save five minutes of their time at Woollies, where they could get everything, instead of $50 of their money. So I had no choice but to close the shop. We continued to provide care and sell mobility equipment from our home office, shipping container and website. During the time, I handed over the management of the business to my niece, April, for about a year while I once again tried to rejuvenate and socialise.

Having had a decent break and now ready to get back to work in 2016, I combined my personal experience with industry best practice along with some new innovative policies.

Having quality care is obviously something everybody would desire, and because I want that for myself and train people accordingly, our clients are able to get a premium human service. While the standard model of care in the industry is to grow the company as big as possible in any one place, resulting in managers managing managers, policies and funding, we developed a sustainable model of quality care for the future. With great pride, we developed a policy of having independent branches with only as many clients as one manger can maintain. It ensured we could deliver a human service and that the manager knows the name of every client, every employee.

Since starting my care company, it has clearly become one of the main purposes of my life. Independence World has often been a source of great joy for me and has many times made me shed a tear. Like when a mother has told me that the carer I trained and sent to her is magic. That their child has never responded to another person like that. And can they please have that carer every day. Words are inadequate to relay the privilege I experience each day. At the moment I have fourteen special people that work in my care company. Some of these people I have known since they were born, some since little children and others that have worked with me multiple times over many years.

Jed has been one of my best friends for twenty-five years now. He has been there for me and taken care of me from the goodness of his heart since the first day I met him. He has also worked for the company a few times taking care of clients. He is a genuine and compassionate being with a heart of gold.

My ex-partner Lucy naturally cared for me when we were together twenty-eight years ago. We have stayed friends and still have great respect for each other. She has recently started managing my Airbnb property. Lucy is the eldest of three sisters that also work in my company.

It was the keen spirit and loyal commitment of this young woman over her first couple of years with me that sparked my desire to start my care company. Katie was my foundation. Even though she has been perpetually five minutes late for the last seventeen years (and owes me therefore in the order of $15,000!), I am happy and humbled to have had her work with me from the beginning.

April is my niece and now the CEO of the company. She has worked for in the company for nine years. She is dedicated and selfless. April is the spitting image of my mum and has the same sweetness and nature. She is also about to become an accountant, and I'm very proud of her. I am blessed to have family to work with and love her dearly.

Belinda has worked for me on and off over the last eleven years and has been a staunch friend. She has endured with me during the worst of times and supported me in every single one of my sometimes outlandish ideas. Her happy dance would encourage anybody to shoot for the moon.

Kirsty threatens to suffocate me, has a wicked sense of humour and laughs at all my jokes so I have kept her around, and she has now worked for me twice in the past eight years. She can't cook but gives a great massage for somebody with a scrawny neck and stick arms.

I have known Dylan for thirty-nine years. As I've already written, he was the manager of my care service once before and did a fantastic job. He is back working for the company again and is a solid and grounding presence. He fills in a care shift if ever needed so our clients never go without support. He is not a great fisherman and his rugby league team is pretty crap, but he is a great soccer coach of his son's team and has a wonderful rapport with our clients and employees alike.

Eden was my live-in carer six years ago before she met a partner and had a little girl, Adeline. Eden enjoys scaring me and has taught Adeline to be a jack-in-the-box from under my bed. Her selfie with me in the background on my belly with the sheets tucked in so I can't move got the most likes on my Facebook page that year. She is now working for me for the second time.

Gina has been my full-time personal carer four times. She has also been fired four times. Each year at our staff party we give away awards for excellence as a disability support worker. We also give away funny awards but they must have two meanings. Last year Gina won the Comeback Award for the quickest and smartest comebacks to the boss but also for coming back the record amount of times after being fired. Behind closed doors she is a marshmallow. She has now been with me for eight years.

Summer is the best cook in town. She has a very motherly instinct, and I always feel safe in her hands. Summer has a can-do attitude, is down to earth and calm in every situation. She is a smart and innovative businesswoman and in the past eleven years she has worked with me twice. I have known her husband for thirty-six years.

Seri is just an awesome person and excellent to party with. Without trying, she outdresses most people. She has a natural trend-setting style, which she seems to be unaware of or rather she just couldn't care about. It means she has no ego even though she is also a brilliant artist. Seri has cared for me a couple of times over the years and is the wife of our company manager, Dylan.

Claire is the youngest of Lucy's sisters, and I have known her since she was just two years old. The sisters would come to our place to watch movies and cartoons. She is my leading disability support worker and an all-round awesome person. Claire is also my main handy person, willing to have a go at anything. She has natural funk and is just groovy. Her confidence and capable nature give me a great sense of security.

When she was just fifteen, Emma travelled with Lucy and me in my truck around Australia as we home-schooled her in little outback towns. Later on in life, Emma was to become a highly paid successful entrepreneur, flying around the world to help organisations develop leadership capability, promote workplace wellbeing and supporting cultural change. Coming home due to the Covid-19 pandemic, I enquired whether she would be interested in doing some consultation for my care company. Emma said that when she read our website, she got goosebumps because we were truly a value-led business making a positive impact in the world. She assumed the role of manager and oversaw our new policies while she inspired our team and tripled our income within six months.

My new executive assistant is Jordyn. She is as sweet as she is polite, intelligent and inspiring. Not to mention way cooler than me. I used to babysit Jordyn when she was just ten years old, when her mother was my carer. Jordyn has impeccable manners and has been my sounding board through the revision of this whole book. Her input has been invaluable. She has an amazingly rich and beautiful voice, a degree in audio and is just awesome with everything music. Together with another couple of brilliant musicians from our company, the sweetest songbird of Vanuatu, Tahni, and our soul brother from the UK, Joe, doing his guitar magic, we have formed our new band, Sweet Island Time.

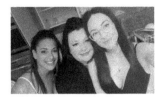

Gina, April, Eden

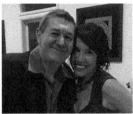

My brother Danny and Belinda

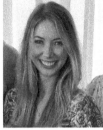

Jordyn

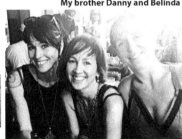

Claire, Emma, Lucy

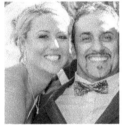

Katie and Paul

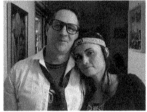

Dylan and Seri

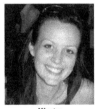

Kirsty

Summer

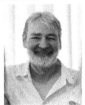

Jed

Happy Paul

After coming back from a holiday in 2019 that included being judged by Peter Rowsthorn, a well-known Australian comedian and actor, for my sit-down comedy, I have gone on writing hundreds of more jokes. The team in my studio are turning them into animations and skits. We're also working on a comedy crime series.

Here are a few of my funnies for people with funny heads. Enjoy:

- Please don't tell your children to not stare at people with disabilities. I was going up in an elevator the other day and a whole family was facing the corner.
- I went on a P&O cruise recently and there were no accessible suites, so I had to have a disabled room. The air conditioner was handicapped, the shower was crippled and the toilet was invalid.

- All the women around me are high maintenance. Jordyn fixes my wheelchair, Gina fixes my bed and Eden fixes my shower chair.
- My carers like to give me s**t. I repaid them last week, twice in my bed and once in my wheelchair.
- I stopped going to church because every time I confessed and had to say a hundred Hail Marys, I always forgot how it started and only could remember, 'Blessed art thou amongst women'.
- What has happened to chivalry? I don't give up my chair for a lady anymore, I never open doors unless they are electric and I always have an excuse for not doing the dishes.
- I feel very discriminated against when I see a disabled parking bay. Why am I always pictured as having a big butt and being white?
- I like to share my inner warmth. So when I am in the shower with my carers, I try to pee on their foot and fart at the same time.

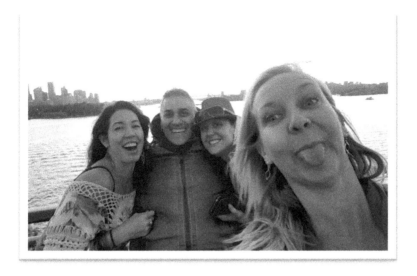

Belinda, Katie and Jo on our comedy trip to Sydney.

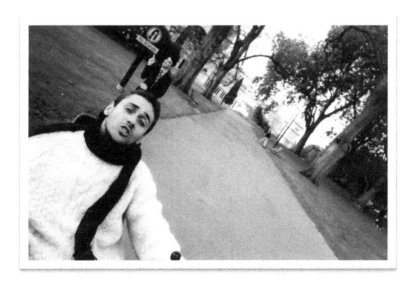

A non-compliance comedian.

The Pursuit of Understanding & Change

…Or Random Stuff to Argue About…

Border Marauders and Power Hoarders (don't mention religion or politics)

Everybody wants to change the world, and I am no different. In my ideal world, there would be no religion. The relationship between us and the universe is just that: Between us and the universe. Everything else that is outwardly expressed about our personal relationship with the universe or God is unique to the individual at different times of their life and can only create division between people.

Companies would have the same law applied to them as governments. Set terms. A period of time for the company to share with the world its product or services, making money and employing people, to ensure the vision of the founder is kept intact. When the appointed time was up, the company would then have to be sold, have its directors newly appointed by the public or simply fold. This would ensure continued innovation and stop environmental rape and monopolies.

All the differences we have as a world of some 200 nations are not as many as the similarities we have or as important as the need to think and act as one world. If we do not act now, we risk the collapse of civilisation; therefore, we must both act as the individual and the world. Not one or the other. If the United Nations were a body where not just nations could vote but every individual on the planet, we might start to see the truth of how all the people of the world really think. Not just that of sometimes corrupt politicians or companies. We can vote as individuals in local, state and national elections. When will we vote as individuals for things that affect us as a world? If you are interested in this subject, please contact admin@theworldvote.world

Financial Support We Can't Abort

With the advent of the National Disability Insurance Scheme in Australia, my life dramatically improved. Worrying about my basic care funding faded and I felt respected as an equal citizen of society. This great new insurance is presently returning $2.25 to every $1 spent on it. When will we honour our aged care system with a similar scheme?

Having a new dignity, and a greater opportunity to contribute to the economy and civilisation, the NDIS has allowed me to achieve many things. One of those is that after many attempts, I have finally been able to finish this book along with many other long-term goals.

Feeling Strong and Taken Wrong

During my many visits to the doctor after my injury, tests showed that I had four and a half times the amount of natural testosterone than that of a normal man. The doctor could not offer any reason for this, so I have had to be aware of the effects that such a high level of this hormone can have. Although it makes me feel very strong in the sense that I intrinsically value integrity, the keeping of my word and the safety of vulnerable or innocent people, it can also easily isolate me from other males. I do, however, have a deep desire to nurture the spirit of all young people, to understand the power of their natural spiritual and emotional strengths, considering keeping the delicate balance of all things in life.

With a Heavy Heart, Do Not Depart

On a number of occasions, the local ABC radio had contacted me regarding my opinion concerning euthanasia or assisted suicide. They had heard that I had a passion for the subject and asked me to speak on air. In general, what I said is that most people would like to have the time to put their affairs in order at the end of their life. They therefore don't want their last few minutes in excruciating pain or in a state where they can't communicate with the people around them and their loved ones.

For some people with certain circumstances, euthanasia or assisted suicide is the only true dignified ending.

In the thirty-four years I have been a quadriplegic, at times I have suffered much physical or psychological pain. The complications surrounding my injury have included muscular, bone or severe nerve pain, regular bladder infections, bladder seizure and hernia, constipation, haemorrhoids, pressure sores, muscle atrophy, violent muscle spasm, insomnia, trialling of a myriad of medications, dysreflexia causing high blood pressure due to a trauma below the injury site, extremely low blood pressure due to poor circulation resulting in fainting and several near-death experiences, and other injury-associated things.

Unfortunately in the earlier days of my injury, these conditions along with lack of physical ability, general public segregation and the psychological effect on me had driven me to the point of contemplating suicide a couple of times. That is of course unlike now. These days I live happily in every moment, for the moment, appreciating every drop of life and being excited for the future.

But for the purpose of this chapter, I would like to say that I have been deeply affected having had a few people in my life commit suicide and a close friend attempting it seven times. Suicide or attempted suicide hurts a large circle of people around the person, for a long time.

In running a care service for fifteen years, I have dealt with many suicidal people and people suffering greatly towards the end of their life.

Education is key and if the topic remains taboo, a high number of people will attempt suicide. However, 85% of people who attempt suicide fail. That failing can have dire consequences including brain damage and the like. People who attempt to hang themselves but do survive without brain damage commonly report that the answer to their problem comes when they are hanging and believe it's too late. They think things like, 'I should have borrowed the money, I should have paid for sex, I should have changed my name, or I should have left the country.' They realise it was emotion that caused them to attempt to take their life. When strong emotions have been let go because they believe that there is now no hope to physically survive, that's when logic kicks in. This is also when your own body fights against the attempt to kill it.

If we come from our emotion, body or mind, we will be limited by the abilities of that aspect of our being. If we come from our spirit, in all things, our power to overcome is limitless.

I Hope My Karma Doesn't Run Over My Dogma

I encourage all people to be aware of having an elitism consciousness. If we believe that God, angels, saints or ascended masters hear our prayers and that we will be graced to have them answered, do we also believe that humans are the lowest rung of consciousness? If not, is it reasonable that animals or demons may be on a lower level and also pray to us? Do we indeed hear them? Do we consider what their prayers are? Do we have the power to, or do we desire to grant them grace?

A family had moved away from their home in Westcourt because the father had been offered a promotion in Melbourne. They had not had time to sell the house and left it in the hands of a local real estate agent. Unbeknownst to the real estate agent, people had broken into the property and were using it for satanic rituals. They had marked a pentagram on the floor and had used it to apparently invite a malevolent entity into the property. The real estate agent managed to sell the property and when the new owners moved in, they began to experience serious problems.

One particular night the entity had become so angry that it picked up their baby and began to throw it against the walls. Beside themselves, they rang the police. The police did not know what to do so in turn rang a local psychic. It seemed that the entity had never been human and therefore conventional means, like that of reasoning or mindfulness, using the power of masters like Jesus, incantations, salts etc., had no bearing on the entity. Having never encountered such a spiritual force, the psychic consulted me. Consulting a couple of powerful friends, and using my spirit-travel ability with all of my knowledge and strength, I was eventually able to move the entity on.

Techniques I have used when dealing with unwanted spiritual entities vary greatly. In some cases, spirits that have been human may have died but not know that they are dead. They can experience death as a long dreamlike state, unaware that their body has passed. If they are disturbing the peace, sometimes just telling them things like that they have passed, what the date is and what is happening in the house or building they are in now can help to free them. I like to tell them that they should turn around and look for a light, which is enough to help some become aware of their reality and move on.

Some others may have passed in a traumatic way and may still be attached to a person, place or thing. In that case, their

ability to physically affect anything in our world is directly re-
lated to the passion, emotion or understanding they have
associated with that person, place or thing. These spirits can
usually be moved on by one or a combination of techniques:
researched reasoning on the actual trauma, relevant affirmations, high notes made by crystals, bells or the like, smoke
from herbs and incense, or chanting the names of gods. However, if the entity has never been human, it may take the
services of people especially astute in the power of spirit, who
may be fearless of having their body possessed or that do not
identify with their physical body as much as an average person.
And these people may need to use their own inner demon to
counteract the opposing force.

Whether we understand it or not, we all have the sweetest
angel and the strongest demon within our own spirit. If we do
not understand this, one or both will always have power over
us.

Experiencing some of these things in life, I have come to
appreciate that our own conscience can create karma, and that
karma can be multi-faceted and sometimes take lifetimes to
realise. The belief in higher powers to forgive us only results in
the diminishment of personal responsibility. Religious and po-
litical dogma is insulting to an infinite universe. May the
universe smack it with its limitless stick.

The Future, The Present & Staying Pleasant

I have written and sung songs since I was a young boy. After my injury I was told that I only have a third of my lung capacity, but I love music and singing so much that forming my band felt natural and inevitable. Songs charm the world for decades like no other thing has ever done. They can influence the world like a subliminal spell more than politics or religion. But more than that for me, music and singing feeds my soul.

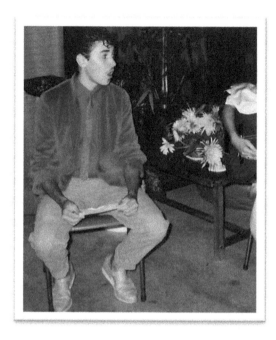

Performing a song I wrote at 18 years old in one of the various communes that I lived in.

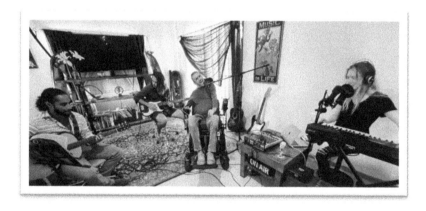

Rehearsing with the band, Sweet Island Time, with Tahni (Silky Bandit), Joe (Nectar Inspector), Paul (Soothe Vigilante) and Jordyn (Sleek Assassin).

234

One of my projects at the time of the publishing of this book is creating another sustainable living community. With everything happening in the world, it seems as though it's the right time again to find a place to nurture my body, mind and spirit with like-minded people.

Unfortunately, even though people want to attempt to be as self-sufficient as possible, governments certainly do not encourage this. I have found that town planning and zoning generally restrict the concept of small freehold parcels of land around a shared ownership parcel unless it is already in an established area, which is not what the people want, nor is it necessarily good for the environment. Governments should learn to understand this basic concept and allow our country to thrive, even in the outback.

Though I advocate for government to allow the creation of small independent communities, I am highly aware of the effects of things like urban sprawl and that for humans to live in harmony with nature we need to have around 44% of the land under conservation. And offsetting carbon emissions is not a solution unto itself in the context of the human footprint and growth in populated areas. We must continue to balance the need for small independent communities with land conservation while continuing to develop our lighter carbon footprint. We must inevitably colonise space and ultimately conquer our ability to travel with our spirit. Should you be interested in this idea, please check out the links and contact page at the end of this book.

Lucid Dreams Are Not What They Seem

Being physically paralysed can be personally confronting to consciousness. As I have lived longer with the injury than without the injury, one would reasonably assume I might be conscious that I am injured or physically restricted when dreaming. But the truth is I am rarely restricted when dreaming. I do not feel any less capable in life than any other man. And this is the consciousness that pervades even my lucid dreams.

I now know that the spirit is the most powerful thing in the universe. Coming from our spirit leads directly to our heart and gives us the right state of mind to be in balance with both the physical and the spiritual worlds. Our relationship with our spirit and the universe has its basis centred on the universe loving us and us loving the universe. When we understand that the spirit is the most powerful thing in the universe, and it is used with a pure intent, all things are possible to it. The only pure intent of our spirit is to be of service to the universe. When we realise this and practise it, we understand that the universe is also in service to our spirit.

This knowledge commands the universe. In the physical world, a person can create a bowl from clay with their hands, a child to stop with a word from our mouths, an event to take place from an initial thought in our head. However, in the astral realm, things are created most powerfully firstly by the spirit, then feelings, thoughts, words, and finally by the physical. The order in which things are created in the astral realm are absolutely the opposite of the order in which things are created in the physical world.

Our spirit body also has form and substance, and it is held together by the passion we have associated with this life. When we look at our skin under a microscope, we see our molecules resonating at a certain speed. So too our spirit body is 'molecules' but made of light, resonating at a higher speed. So fast in fact that it is in most cases invisible, or we can see through the spirit body. The greater the strength of our attachment, the slower our light molecules resonate, therefore allowing our spirit to have subsequent physical influence in the real world.

Through time I came to realise that to free my spirit, I had to be in the right mind space. I worked out that for me, this came through conscious or lucid dreaming. From that deep state of alpha thought, I envisaged a way that I could force my spirit free and into the astral world. I also devised a way that I could bring back scientific proof for myself – physical and tangible evidence.

I would give myself a 'mission'. Something that I could re-member and then check on when I was awake. I closed my eyes and opened a book at a random page. I then put the book beside me and closed my eyes to sleep. My mission was to travel in my spirit and look at the page number and then recall the page number when I awoke without opening my eyes. As this mission was to eventually take many months, I had some-body put the book facing upwards on top of my wardrobe. You could also have somebody write a number on a piece of paper for you and stick it somewhere on top of something high, facing upwards.

As mentioned, I did eventually conquer my spirit and taught people how to travel in their own spirit, meeting them face to face in the astral world. I know there is no greater thing that I can share with this world. Therefore, as much as it is able to be explained in words, I give my readers the follow-ing:

After we close our eyes, we usually see one or more of a number of things. We may see the refraction of light left over from the last thing that we were looking at. We could see patches of colour on a dark background. Sometimes we see a mandala, a pattern whereby the beginning and end are the same, and endless. We might also purpose to visualise some-thing. If we are trying to sleep, we might see scenes from the movie that our mind is making. If we are actually falling asleep, we enter a level of consciousness that science calls the 'hypnogogic' state. I learned that we can allow any of these things, or a dream itself, to be a doorway into a state of conscious dreaming.

One night I dreamed that I was in the bathroom of my childhood home, but the walls were made of newspaper. When I woke the next morning, I asked myself, 'Why didn't I know that I was dreaming? The walls of the bathroom of my childhood home weren't really made of newspaper!' That is an initial step, asking yourself or your subconscious, the question regarding your ability to lucid dream. I say subconscious because our brains are in the alpha state last thing at night or first thing in the morning, making those times naturally easier to program our subconscious to perform an outcome.

That night I posed the question again, humbly asking 'God' in prayer to allow me to realise that I am dreaming when I am asleep. Then with the voice of God, I affirmed it, 'I know when I am dreaming when I am asleep,' repeating it with a loud, resonating resolve. It was enough to prompt me when I indeed fell asleep and began to dream. I found myself once again in my old bathroom with the walls made of newspaper. Upon such realisation, the scene started to dissolve. The reason for this is that when we become conscious that we are dreaming, emotion arises due to the exciting prospects it brings. We can fly and do otherwise impossible things.

This emotion is magnified in dreams and often activates the adrenaline gland in the physical body, which will only release so much but then in turn begins to dissolve the scene and wakes up the physical body from the dream, usually with a jolt. If the adrenaline gland is activated by joy or fear, excitement or anxiety, it is enough to ruin your dream or meditative state. One must avoid this by immediately grounding oneself in that particular consciousness. This can be achieved by sitting down, focusing on the breath, calming the emotion and using balancing affirmations such as Be, Stillness, I Am, or by chanting. This will solidify the scene.

Next, you will need to control your mind from wandering. Focus on the intent you have for being there with unwavering attention. What is your mission? Even a slight stray in this consciousness can have unintended consequences. When we have our eyes open, our consciousness is telling us everything that is going on around us while our subconscious may be in the background, talking or singing etc. But when we have our eyes closed, we are the conscious mind in the middle while our subconscious is what we are seeing manifest all around us, in our mind. Here, we begin our co-creation with the universe.

Our subconscious is created by our intention or expectation. It is also magnified: fear a dragon and 1000 can appear. Remain calm and you will be Alice in Wonderland. Frequently, we are other characters in our dreams and other times just an observer. For instance, you may have been born with a different name than what you have at present. So, remember just focus on working out your mission – the page number. So how do you do that? One way is to look for clues about the date that you are dreaming. If you can somehow work out what date it is in your dream, you will also remember who you are and where you are at the same time. This triangulates your consciousness into the understanding of being actually asleep but aware of the body in real-time. If you can't, just focus on the number.

If you are able to achieve this, your mind is in alpha and you should find it easy to remain relaxed. This is when you can try to travel from your body in your spirit. Some people attempt to float upwards but sitting up is more natural. Try to ever so gently sit up in the bed. If you go too fast, you will wake up your physical body. Again, it took me months to master just this one step. It really is akin to tricking your body into staying still while you emerge from an ocean. A limited ocean of ignorance into the limitless sky of eternity.

When you first sit up and look at your physical body, you will remember that the spirit is the real you, the eternal you, the limitless you. You will remember that your physical experience is temporary and very short. You will understand that all physical, mental, emotional or social trauma experienced in your physical body has no effect or bearing on your indestructible eternal spirit. You will begin to conquer your fears, anxieties and weaknesses and the things of the body. The world, power, fame, materialism and death start to fade in the all-empowering reach and understanding of your spirit.

As you begin to spend time in your spirit, you will start to understand that there are no problems. You will experience omniscience, knowing all things; omnipresence, being anywhere or everywhere at the same time; and omnipotence, able to do any and all things. You will experience existence as one, the blanket understanding and acceptance of all things as they are.

Though you will begin to understand how important it is to spend time as your pure spirit, you will also understand how precious and important it is to get the most out of your physical life. You will probably appreciate it more and be more practical. What do you call your eternal self? Your earthly name? You will remember that your earthly name is just for one lifetime.

Eternal truth is undeniably recognisable. If we go through a whole lifetime not remembering our eternal truth, we sometimes forget our temporary purpose.

Many people do astral travel already in the night during their dreams. Unfortunately, they simply do not remember the experience. One reason for this is because of a limited grasp of what memory is. A doctor tells us that every cell in our body, right down to the retina in our eye and the marrow in our bones, is replaced every seven years. Yet most scars on our bodies remain permanent. This is because memory is not confined to the organ of the brain. The whole body retains memory.

Scientists have recently discovered that by connecting our body to a certain computer sensor, the monitor will show that we also have an outer membrane or electro-magnetic body. It is this area where the fragile and subtle memories of travel in the astral realm are kept. On waking we tend to open our eyes, stretch and move, thus consequentially we fracture it and disperse it into fragments, making it harder, yet not impossible to recall. If we are to simply become aware, be conscious, realise that we are awake, and reverse our thoughts, one by one, without moving, we are able to remember our travels in the astral realm. It is then that we can implement the power and understanding of our spirit in the waking and physical world.

Because the spirit has the ability to be omnipresent, it means that if entering the astral realm without a single strong purpose or intent, the spirit may go many places at once, thus making all those experiences harder to recall upon waking and to put into practice in the physical world.

Unfortunately, most people are more afraid of their own, other people's and the universe's destructive powers than they are appreciative of creative or positive powers. Therefore, they shy away from spirit travel in the astral realm. I reassure you that the bad things in existence are very much outweighed by the good.

The love and joy that we experience as humans only begins to prepare us for what lies ahead. The pain or suffering that we may have experienced physically, mentally, emotionally or socially in the past is only meant to help us to appreciate our true eternal reality in the present.

It is my hope that you learn to travel this earth and the realms beyond in your spirit without the need to use green-house gases. That you journey to other worlds, learn knowledge kept secret or inaccessible, seek the wisdom behind your soul's earthly incarnation or karma, talk with loved ones present or passed, seek out angels, guides, saints or ascended masters and grasp the truth about how your body, mind, soul and spirit work together. That you can become a catalyst for change by speaking to people from your spirit who are influential or famous (they do hear you). That you advocate for freedom and justice and even fight and douse with light actual other-dimensional demons. You do not have to wait to become enlightened or an angel, you can do the work of the angels, right now, and whisper in the ears of children to give them hope.

May you find peace in knowing and experiencing that infinite power and freedom of spirit is your eternal truth.

My Best Mate

My life has truly been a pendulum swing from one extreme to the other. I have tried to write this book many times over the past thirty years or so but one thing or another has always stopped me. I have many more stories to tell, though this book must end somewhere. Before this one does though, I must pay tribute to my best mate: my mum. Mum was my rock, but she passed away in early December 2017. If she hadn't been by my side, my whole life would have been very different. I give honour to a woman that would do everything she could for me until her passing at the age of eighty-two.

Mum, it was always you and me against the world. I loved your happy-dance jig and pirouette. You were the best cuppa tea and bakies maker ever. It seems like not long ago at all that I would listen for the sound of your door rolling back in the morning and hear the shuffle of your slippers while I waited for you to appear in one of a number of cute, cosy-looking dressing gowns with our cups of tea. Your voice was always sweet and calm, saying good morning to me. You always asked me how I slept and were interested in everything I had to say and was doing. Then you would waddle off again for your crosswords and coffee. We looked forward to our Saturday punt and footy game. We had many a wild night. We had many a tear. I miss your soft skin and my kiss goodnight. I love you to the moon and the stars and back.

My mum was a genuine champion in many ways. She could laugh and swear with the best of them. Her love and devotion had given me the motivation and inspiration to live as full a life as I feel I've been blessed to have had.

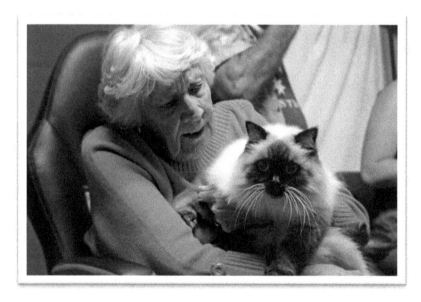

My best mate, my Mum.

A Delight to Write…Not My Last Chapter

Curiously, my injury has caused me suffering but also presented joyful experiences that I would not have otherwise had.
Children see me as no threat and freely smile at me, often
starting conversations they ordinarily would not have with a
stranger. Seeing me in a wheelchair, they know I pose no
physical danger. It means that every time I go out, people
from all walks of life actually try to catch my eye. They hope
to impart some joy, some acknowledgment. The delight I get
when our passing eyes catch, and I get a smile, extends from
toddlers to shy teenagers, wild-looking adolescents, burly men
and the aged. They all try to relate somehow. It is truly beautiful and one of the greatest blessings in my life. In that
moment, we acknowledge the gift of life itself, there is mutual

respect, compassion, and we see each other's souls. It brings healing and humanity to both of us.

Having had the pleasure of being cared for by a great number of diverse people over a long period of time, I feel qualified to say that the true nature of a human is compassionate and selfless. It is behind closed doors, when there is just a carer and myself, that I have seen this over and over again. And as we explore science and have begun to understand the seeming limitlessness of inner and outer space, we have also begun to appreciate our real nature, giving hope to humanity, peace and oneness in our world.

I also feel compelled to say that though my injury has left me very physically restricted, I have throughout time, learned to still enjoy my body.

The restriction of the injury has though, at times, forced me to confront myself in ways that I believe I would not have considered otherwise. I have felt compelled to pose deep questions regarding not only my injury but existence itself. Given enough time and the right circumstances, I believe that any lateral-thinking adult would eventually contemplate these questions. In modern times though, our lives demand so much attention that we have forgotten to ask the important questions. But if we do not ask these questions, and in some cases, have some sort of answer, then society, science, religion or somebody else will answer them for us. And most of the time, asking the question is more important than having an answer. Give yourself the time to ask the big questions.

Over the years when young people have expressed to me that they did not know what they wanted to do with their life, sometimes I have said to ask themselves what they wanted to do with their death? They mostly think that is a morbid or negative subject to consider. But I tell them that in fact, most people live their whole life according to what they hope happens in the last few moments. They have an unrealistic vision that they will know when they are dying, their family and friends will be around them and they will have time to make peace with themselves, their maker and be ready for their journey to the next dimension or reincarnation et cetera.

In truth, even if we did know when the last day or few minutes of our life was going to be, most times those around us are not aware enough to not interfere in the end processes and are thinking about their coming grief, their inheritance, what they should say on social media and sometimes other negative things. So why do old dogs go off into the bush if they think they are dying? Because as the Buddhists say, the time of your death is more important than the time of your birth. It is the accumulation of everything that has happened over your lifetime; it's not just about the one event of your birth.

What I do encourage people to consider is giving themselves an estimate of their life span. And a vision of how they hoped to be living when that time comes. Then their spirit has a goal for this life. A path to take, so their spirit can give them signs that they are making the right decisions. They will feel a sense of achievement and that they are following their own destiny.

Our soul is individual and free, there can be none alike; otherwise, there is no freedom.

Only in the stillness of heart does the ocean of emotion cease. Only in the void of nothingness is there peaceful meditation. Only when the mind and soul have no desire for a moment, the abyss of bliss emerges, the remembrance of eternal freedom. Now, I am like a bird whose claws are locked on its perch, it knows that it is free, it has spread its wings in anticipation of flight, but it has been petrified in part and can't let go for fears of losing its world. But soon I will return to the earth's floor and become dust again. I will return to the elements that created me. I will quickly forget my previous name and remember my eternal truth. Just that I am eternal. Without name, without body, without limit. I will evaluate my life and ponder its greatest lessons and experiences. I will wander alone, drawing in the peace of the loud silence. I will sit in silent awe of the beauty of the universe. I will once again be the observer, choosing not to interact with the physical worlds, for an aeon or two.

Every time you meditate, you realise how important it is. It releases suppressed emotion. It puts priorities in order. It allows the time needed to visualise your future dreams. It is an actual escape from the world. It allows peace of mind. It improves memory. You can hear your own voice above everything else in the world again. You become present and in the moment.

These next sentences are from other people but were profound enough to me to remember always:

Don't condemn the smoke that has got us this far, to here, where we are; bless and magnify the goodness of the air.

We can afford all things except waste.

Never compromise your strength for an ideal.

Peace and perfection are the milestones of love.

All is fair in love and war.

Have one master or have everything as your master.

I have seen all manner of miracles in my life. Things that are unexplainable. This is not a mundane world. There is such thing as real magic. We can create our destiny. We can change anything. Our spirit and its power to create is boundless. We must come from our spirit. Our spirit is already free. Already at peace.

To save ourselves, those that we love and our planet, we must protect what we know and what we have.

Love creates all things. The universe is manifested through love – self-love and selfless love.

Love is sacred and limitless. Its eternal truth is unconditional.

Life is conceived by love and is sustained by love.

Anybody can do anything they can imagine in this world. Will you let life and circumstance make or break you? I say let existence shower you with the richness and eternal abundance of the universe. May my readers be challenged and inspired to enjoy the infinite freedom and strength of their own spirit, yet buoyed and empowered by my spirit and life.

I had the honour of being asked by the Human Rights Commission of Queensland to be in the first group of people in Cairns to become 'Living Books' for International Human Rights Day. As part of the presentation at the Cairns Regional Art Gallery we were asked to speak on ABC radio. Having been interviewed by the ABC a few times previously, I had performed some of my poems. I know that people don't generally remember whole poems, only the gist or maybe one line. So, to end my book, I have written some one-line poems that can be remembered when we need strength of mind, heart and spirit:

Natural instinct cannot be taught, so trust yourself and first thought.

No trouble you find is worth peace of mind.

Whatever the fact, it's how you react.

Life's no race, use poise and grace.

Don't be affected; stay cool, calm and collected.

In alarm, breathe, be calm.

Endure the length with courage, with strength.

In the midst of rigour, remember your vigour.

Don't just fold, be strong, be bold.

Save regret and need of healing, use your sense and gut feeling.

Your words are your power; they can make sweet what was sour.

Whether devil or angel relay it, it's simply how you say it.

Let no fool break your cool.

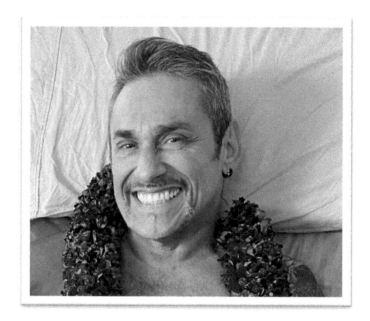

Acknowledgements

Acknowledgement must go to my many family members, friends and carers that endured countless drafts of this book during the past 30 years.

I sincerely thank Jordyn Harpur for all her valuable insight and humble but honest and constructive criticism during the latest review over the past 12 months.

I'd like to give thanks to Luke Cuthbertson for the countless hours he put into the film clips and animation for the presentation of this book. Thank you to the many people that gave their written permission to be included in my stories.

I also highly appreciate having found such a wonderful person as Dr Juliette Lachemeier of The Erudite Pen as my editor extraordinaire, finding that she not only provided a wonderful and professional service, but she had a passion and praise that energised me and inspired me to put my whole soul and mind into this work. I felt privileged to have Juliette offer to publish this, my first book, and now, and in large part thanks to Juliette, I am already starting on my second.

ABOUT THE AUTHOR

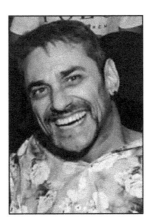

Paul Innes was born in Darlinghurst, Sydney, but now lives in
the tropical paradise of Cairns, Far North Queensland. He began an acting career before sustaining a spinal injury while
swimming in Kuranda at age twenty that caused quadriplegia.
After founding a rights incorporation for people with disabilities, Paul also went on to become a founding committee
member of a number of community organisations.

Paul developed a sustainable self-sufficient community that eventually became home to four of Queensland's missing frogs and the site of Australia's first Rainbow Gathering. He is currently searching for the next property that he will develop as a resort-style sanctuary.

Thirty-four years later, Paul Innes is a holder of two Guinness Book of World Records and teaches astral travel. He opened his own disability care service, Independence World, which now runs independently of him. He spends time writing and filming as a sit-down comedian and recording with his band Sweet Island Time.

Enjoyed the book? You can contact the author at:

Email: director@independenceworld.com.au

Facebook – Sustainable Living Sanctuary:
https://www.facebook.com/groups/4502560093167212

Facebook – Independence World:
https://www.facebook.com/independenceworld.com.au/

Website: www.independenceworld.com.au

The World Vote: admin@theworldvote.world

If you liked the book, please leave a review on Amazon,
Goodreads or with the author directly. Reviews are invaluable
in supporting an author's hard work
and are greatly appreciated.

CPSIA information can be obtained
at www.ICGtesting.com
Printed in the USA
BVHW012050091222
653835BV00022B/555

9 780645 600506